"With rare and disarming candour, Pietro Roberto Goisis narrates both his patients' stories and his own experience as a psychoanalyst, revealing how therapists too are changed by the patients they care for."

Micol Artom, *User Research Lead, NHS*

"Moving between reflection, memory, and clinical vignette, the book evokes the quiet drama of analytic work and the delicate human stories that unfold within it."

William Glover, *Past-President, American Psychoanalytic Association*

"This book will speak to psychoanalysts and psychotherapists at every stage of practice, affirming the quiet complexity of our work and the enduring importance of holding a space where transformation can occur."

Alessandra Lemma, *Visiting Professor, Psychoanalysis Unit, UCL and Fellow, British Psychoanalytic Society*

"Here is a psychoanalyst who talks about his work without idealization or defensiveness, minimizing theory. He conveys his idea of psychoanalysis to us: a mutually transformative experience, imperfect and deeply human."

Vittorio Lingiardi, *Psychiatrist and Psychoanalyst, Sapienza University of Rome, 'The Sigourney Award 2023' Recipient*

A Psychoanalyst and His Patients

A Psychoanalyst and His Patients offers an intimate and authentic glimpse into the analytic room, revealing transformative encounters between psychoanalyst and patient through vivid clinical vignettes.

Pietro Roberto Goisis conveys the living reality of psychoanalytic work, where words, silences, emotions and everyday details become the raw material for healing and growth. Through compelling narratives spanning adolescent identity crises, trauma recovery, sexual exploration and despair, Goisis demonstrates how the analytic space becomes a crucible for meaning-making and transformation. Each chapter illuminates not only the patients' journeys but also the analyst's own vulnerability and evolution, showing how psychoanalysis is fundamentally a shared human experience where fragmented experiences find coherence and dark territories are welcomed and reworked. This book bridges the gap between clinical practice and accessible storytelling, making the complexity of psychoanalysis comprehensible without sacrificing depth or rigour. Written with poetic sensitivity yet clinical precision, this book reveals the analytic room not as a mysterious or abstract space, but as a living environment capable of welcoming and transforming all who enter it.

It will be of great interest to psychoanalysts in practice and in training, mental health professionals, students of psychology and counselling, and to readers interested in therapeutic practice.

Pietro Roberto Goisis is a psychiatrist, psychotherapist and psychoanalyst based in Italy, and a past member of the Italian Psychoanalytic Society (SPI) and an IPA-approved Child and Adolescent Psychoanalyst. He has been also Adjunct Professor at the Catholic University of Milan. He is the author of multiple books on psychoanalysis, including (with Angelo Antonio Moroni) *Psychoanalytic Diaries of the Covid-19 Pandemic* (Routledge).

A Psychoanalyst and His Patients

A Room for Dreams, Hopes and Desires

Pietro Roberto Goisis

Routledge
Taylor & Francis Group
LONDON AND NEW YORK

Designed cover image: Anna Resmini

First published 2027
by Routledge
4 Park Square, Milton Park, Abingdon, Oxon OX14 4RN

and by Routledge
605 Third Avenue, New York, NY 10158

Routledge is an imprint of the Taylor & Francis Group, an informa business

The soundtrack for the book is available on a Spotify playlist.

You can listen to it by typing www.bit.ly/nellastanzadeisogni

British Library Cataloguing in Publication Data
A catalogue record for this book is available from the British Library

ISBN: 978-1-041-28354-6 (hbk)
ISBN: 978-1-041-28353-9 (pbk)
ISBN: 978-1-003-75903-4 (ebk)

DOI: 10.4324/9781003759034

Typeset in Times New Roman
by Taylor & Francis Books

To Emma and Bianca
To Gherardo
α and ω

Contents

Acknowledgements

The people I met. Those who entered my room. Those mentioned in the book. For agreeing to be there.

My colleagues and friends.

The readers.

Anna Resmini for the gift of the cover illustration. Arialdo for the soundtrack.

Camilla Amadei for the affectionate concession of Gherardo's writing.

Giorgia Benusiglio and family for sharing the pain.

Legnano, London, Milan, Rozzano, Trieste, Garda Lake, the Aosta Valley, Umbria.

Deserts, journeys, races, walks.

Enrico Damiani Editore e Associati, the Italian publisher.

Routledge – Taylor & Francis Group, the English publisher.

Alice and Tommaso for the implicit power of generativity and passing on.

Cristina for her support, stolen time, patience, waiting. And love. Love for care, the care of love.

Franco Battiato for *La Cura*. Because we are all special beings to be cared for.

Ivano Fossati, because *We have time*. A time to sow and a time to wait for the harvest. A time to dream and a time for dreaming.

Preface

It is a pleasure to introduce the English edition of *A Psychoanalyst and His Patients. A Room for Dreams, Hopes and Desires.* From the first pages, Pietro Roberto Goisis invites us into the intimate world of the consulting room – a place that, for many of us, becomes almost a second home. What struck me immediately is the honesty and simplicity with which he writes about his work. There is no grandiosity here, no attempt to impress. Instead, Goisis reveals the small and often ordinary moments through which deep change can occur. His attention to these moments, and to the people who bring their lives into his room, makes this a book that both clinicians and lay readers can appreciate.

What Goisis offers is not a manual, nor an argument for a particular school of psychotherapy. Rather, it is a meditation on what happens when two human beings sit together and try to make sense of suffering, hope and the desire to live differently. He writes openly about his own anxieties, mistakes and hesitations – experiences every therapist knows well but that we rarely speak about. In doing so, he reminds us that our work is sustained not by flawless technique but by presence, curiosity and the willingness to be moved and changed by our patients.

I was especially touched by the central motif of the room. For Goisis, the consulting room is not simply an office but a living space that evolves with each person who enters it. It is shaped by history – his and theirs – and by the shared task of finding meaning in moments that can be joyful, painful, confusing or transformative. Readers will recognise in his descriptions the delicate choreography of psychotherapy: the anticipation of the waiting room, the first glance between therapist and patient, the ritual of beginning, the surprising directions a session can take when we allow ourselves to be guided by genuine contact.

The clinical vignettes – rendered with grace and compassion – reveal an analyst who loves his work and the people who entrust him with their stories. Whether he is working with a woman grieving lost pregnancies, an adolescent navigating fragility and defiance or a patient whose despair narrows the horizon of the possible, Goisis finds meaning in gestures, silences, missteps and unexpected creativity. His accounts of adolescents are particularly compelling. They illustrate how much courage it takes for young people to approach therapy and how vital it is that we meet them with authenticity rather than pretence. Throughout the book, Goisis demonstrates that therapy is not a set of procedures but a relationship that unfolds over time, requiring patience, humility and an openness to being changed by the encounter.

English-speaking readers will find much to appreciate here: a lyrical sensibility, a deep humanism and a reminder of why many of us entered this field in the first place. *A Psychoanalyst and His Patients. A Room for Dreams, Hopes and Desires* is an invitation to slow down and trust the subtle processes that occur when two people sit together, listen carefully and search for truth. Goisis repeatedly shows us something I have long asserted: this undertaking is not for the faint of heart!

I am grateful that this book is now available to a wider audience. I believe it will resonate with clinicians who value the relational and experiential dimensions of psychotherapy, as well as with readers who simply want to understand what makes these encounters meaningful.

Stephen E. Finn, Ph.D.
Founder and President Center for Therapeutic Assessment, Austin, Texas, USA
Clinical Associate Professor, University of Texas at Austin, USA

1 The Room

I love psychoanalysis, this psychoanalysis.
I love my work.
I continue to do it every day,
every month, every year.
I don't want to stop.
I hope I can keep doing this
as long as someone sits down in front of me,
asks me something, and I can give them an answer.
It's my life. Part of it.

Pietro Roberto Goisis, 2018

Claudia, a young woman, had called me on the phone. She had insisted on seeing me even though I had told her I was unavailable. She was pregnant. Happy, but scared at the same time. In recent years, two pregnancies had ended suddenly and painfully, one shortly after the other. She feared for the current one. She had already had a psychoanalytic experience in the past, which had also been traumatic in some respects. She said she spent more than a year on the couch, twice a week, in total silence, both she and the analyst. During that time, she said she couldn't ask for a change nor had the courage to end it. She was wary about asking for help again. At the same time, she felt the need for emotional support during her pregnancy, however it could go. She was intelligent, pleasant and narcissistically convinced that she would be able to convince me to make an exception for her notwithstanding my lack of time. And she continued to oscillate between the desire to put herself on the line again and the fear that it caused her. She had already strongly invested in the child she was expecting, as if it were already born, from the way she talked about it.

In the end, we both broke our hesitation and began therapy.

A few months later, she reminded me of the exact moment when something truly important had happened.

We were at the end of one of our first meetings.

"I think coming here is the first good thing I've done for my baby," she said (and it took a considerable effort for her to open like that).

DOI: 10.4324/9781003759034-1

I replied with a question: "Why don't you think of this as the first thing your baby has done for you?"

It was that simple shift in perspective that made her fall in love with our work together: in a single sentence, it confirmed that she was loved, that her unborn child really existed, and it was the first snapshot of her with her son, together. He was born on time and is doing well. He was soon followed by a little brother.

Things that can happen and only happened to me there, in that place. Just as without a tennis court Andre Agassi would never have existed, if there were no room there would be no therapist, no patients. Sometimes I even feel that it is magical, that it brings out the best in me, something I didn't even know I had, that I couldn't find anywhere else, that surprises me.

As children, our room is the centre of our world, where we are initially somewhat confined. We receive the invitation, sometimes the order, to "Go to sleep!", that can make us feel excluded from the adult world. Then, from early adolescence onwards, our room becomes an inaccessible fortress which we jealously defend. No matter what happens inside, no one is allowed to enter, and no one is allowed to rummage through bags, drawers, diaries, backpacks or bookcases.

The concept of a world apart also pervades the place where therapist and patient meet. What "really" happens there is one of the mysteries and curiosities of both professionals and people who have never entered and who, perhaps, one day might. Parents who struggle from asking: "How did it go? What did you talk about?" Spouses or partners who glance sideways at their partner in the hope of catching a clue, almost grasping for some kind of revelation. Ordinary people who know nothing but say a lot. And the room, an entity, remains, somewhat haughtily, observing the whirlwind of thoughts that it is destined to harbour.

For those of us who are therapists, the room represents a goal, an objective, the confirmation of an identity.

Young colleagues in training call it "the studio". They talk about it for days on end, comparing notes, evaluating notices and advertisements, feeding off word of mouth. They wait for the right moment. Patiently. More or less.

When they finally manage to rent one, the next immediate inevitable desire becomes buying their own place. So, their office or "studio" rented, shared or subdivided, even if only for half a day a week, begins to offer the sweet taste of a profession that is taking the form of something tangible or better yet real. Sometimes, we can have our practice set up but there are no patients yet. It doesn't matter. In any case, if we didn't have a room, even a temporary set-up even in their own home, there could be no patients.

"Two People Talking in a Room" is the wonderful title of the article written in 1984 by the analyst Luciana Nissim, which conveys the most human, authentic and truthful image of what happens in this place.

A place where anything can happen. The room of dreams, for real.

When we move into a house, we immediately feel the need to renovate it, so that it truly becomes ours.

Significant and unexpected renovations take place in the "dream room". Renovations can occur in our interlocutors and oftentimes in us as well. And as in any respectable renovation, there are always unexpected events and extra work. The fundamental principle is to respect the basic elements and substance of the space in question, being careful to avoid distorting its spirit and identity. Whatever happens the room is always there to permit it, guarantee, protect, and bear witness to it.

It welcomes and hosts those who decide to enter it. I often wonder how they got there. How many questions did they ask themselves or others? How much research did they do on the internet? How many phone calls did they imagine or attempt?

I am there, in my room.

It's comfortable, whether it's warm or cool, sunny or raining outside.

I am there, waiting.

I know that whoever arrives has travelled along roads, used transportation, maybe struggled to find the time.

Who enters the room? How can we define them? Well, first and foremost, as people. That's how they arrive. That is already a lot. Then, as I believe they know, the moment they cross the threshold, they become "patients". This can be a pleasant transition, accompanied by a feeling of anticipation.

Or it can be painful and difficult to accept, so much so, that sometimes months or even years pass before they manage to become patients. If they manage to do so.

And I am always there.

My room holds me, defines me, supports me and becomes my accomplice.

Long before it became "my" playground, it was a place that I frequented when I was the patient, for my own personal analysis.

I had started seeing a therapist a few months earlier: I was engaged, motivated, happy. That day I was late, and I felt bad about it. It was only a few minutes, but for me it meant wasting precious time. Come to think of it, I wasn't thinking about her – the therapist – at all, the person who was waiting for me – or who knows, maybe she was minding her own business? – I was preoccupied with myself, with traffic, parking, the things I had to say that had been stressing me since the night before. Only one single event separated my early Thursday morning session, that I was late for, from the previous one on Wednesday evening: the ritual tennis match with my father.

I have often thought that there was no event more symbolic, at that stage of my life and my analysis, than a frank and masculine confrontation between a father and a son. We had always had less trouble with yellow tennis balls than with words. The latter were difficult and stunted, the former rolling and piercing. We gave each other a good thrashing in an hour of fierce exchanges. I could never beat him, but we ended the game exhausted and happy. I think he was satisfied in continuing confirmation of his supremacy, and if we leave Oedipus out of the whole thing, I was grateful to spend time with him. Gratefully happy that it was just the two of us.

That morning, as often happened, I was about to spill out my dreams and recount the latest episode of an endless challenge that the tennis match had triggered – I felt like one of the protagonists of *The Duellists* by Ridley Scott.

I was late, it's true, but not "too late"; I was sure my analyst wouldn't mind, nor comment on my delay. I finally found a good parking space – "Lucky break", I thought – locked the car quickly with the remote car key, and then ran, rapidly leaping up the stairs. Almost like the hero in a video game, I hurdled through all the doors: the gate, front door, small door, antechamber, and luckily the door to the room was open. I passed through it too and threw myself onto the couch. I made it. Deep sigh.

Only then did I notice that she, the analyst, was standing there, next to the desk. She was munching on something and looking at me in amazement. I remember that the window was open. She calmly closed it, swallowed the last bite, approached the couch and sat down in the armchair behind me. I will omit the sequence of precise and timely interpretations that she poured over me, caused by that dive into the room.

I hadn't stopped in the waiting room, I hadn't waited for her to come and show me in.

It was true, in fact, I felt that that room was mine alone, no matter who else was there. That time slot of the session was mine alone, despite my delay. That place was mine. She was little more than an intruder.

We seek relationships intensely; we suffer when they end or never start. We need to feel the benevolent and welcoming presence of those who are with us. We experience deep feelings of abandonment and loss when our interlocutors fail us. We want words and comfort.

Then, sometimes, it is enough for us to be in that space, the space of the room, as if it were a hyperbaric capsule launched into space. We inhabit it, we make it our own, we seem to get lost in time.

How can such an experience of "deprivation", as some describe it – "My therapist never talks!" – become therapeutic and transformative?

For me, as a patient, it was magical, unique and unrepeatable. The feeling that something that had never happened before was happening now and would never happen again. It doesn't matter who you are, who she or he is, whether you are there for money or love, interest or work. It is difficult to experience and remember moments that can be so intense, exclusive and special. Apart from marriage, the birth of children and painful losses.

We were talking about the room. My room. Or rather, the rooms.

Above the wall telephone – landline – in the house where I grew up, a sheet torn from a squared notebook was stuck to the wall. It contained the telephone numbers of my temporary and initial places of work. My mother's unmistakable handwriting updated the list, adding new numbers from time to time. She stopped at the sixth line. There were too many, she had had enough.

The first room, when I was a specialist trainee and did my internship (now called a traineeship) in the women's section of a psychiatric ward, was a bed.

During the morning "rounds", the procession of doctors – head physician, assistant, assistants, specialists, interns, as well as nurses – used to go from room to room and assess the care. When a student like me had to talk to one of the three patients assigned to him in a room, he had no choice but stand by the side of one of the beds, maybe pull up a chair or perch on the edge of the mattress, if the patient gave him permission, and especially if the conversation promised to be long. I wonder if my relational style could have been influenced by this forced intimacy.

Looking back now, I always recall a feeling of mutual fatigue, perhaps embarrassment. Extreme disparity reigned between us: one of us was a hospital patient, wearing pyjamas and, at best, a dressing gown, the other was strutting around in his starched white coat, with a badge on his lapel bearing his name written in marker pen. However, I am convinced that it is also thanks to these conflicting emotions that I learned my trade and use it wherever needed and however attempted.

An alternative to the ward's bedrooms? The dining room.

Of course, only until the tables were set. Then the interviews ended.

A promotion was being able to use the ward's cloakroom for meetings with my patients. It was small and private, with two armchairs placed there for that purpose.

The only problem was that the nurses could suddenly appear, who were both surprised and amused, looking for linen to change the beds.

I remember that room being the scene of a somewhat surreal conversation: a patient had great difficulty relating to men and tended to avoid any contact with them. So, I launched into a kind of speech.

"It seems to me that you judge men using the same criteria you would use for a field of carrots: it's true that at first glance they all look the same, only the green part sticks out, but you can only assess their quality and goodness by pulling them out of the ground. It seems to me that you are refusing to eat any carrots at all just to avoid those few that are no good, perhaps you could try judging the carrot only after you have picked it!"

I honestly don't remember the patient's reaction, apart from a certain perplexity at my symbolically imprudent metaphor. In any case, despite so much time having passed, that episode still comes to mind even today and evokes tenderness for my rather clumsy and naïve therapeutic effort.

Later, the room in the Local Public Services would arrive.

Of course, it was obviously better than a bed or a storeroom, but I still had to share it with other colleagues, who outnumbered the available rooms. It was difficult to personalise a space that everyone used in their own way, with different tastes and needs. At this point, it was idealistically defined as a neutral place, but unfortunately it was closer to anonymous, if not outright squalor.

This is why I believe that, while waiting for "a room of my own", I decided to use the on-call room in the private clinic as if it were mine. It was my first paying job. I am somewhat embarrassed to confess that it was a bedroom once again, but it was a comfortable refuge, with a television and minibar, where I could rest and wait until they called me. It was a sort of base camp, refuge and recharge station all in one.

The rooms where most of the work was done, were the well-furnished and comfortable single rooms of the hospitalised patients.

So, once again, bedrooms were the only places where the interviews were possible.

It seems like I had really seen it all! Patients arriving in the middle of the night, acute crises, tantrums and oddities. And even a few tragedies.

In my own small way, I visited an interactive and *evolving* museum of psychiatry during those years. Renowned psychoanalysts; pioneers in the treatment of psychosis; the last shocking but "decisive" electroshock treatments under anaesthesia; the first heroin addicts; experimenters with new deadly cocktails of multiple substances; therapeutic communities; alcoholics' groups; modern-day pathologies, including intriguing and unsettling borderline cases and identity crises, and disorienting, incomprehensible and elusive eating disorders. I had encounters with a big part of humanity that was suffering, indifferently composed of individuals who were either likeable and tender or aggressive and contemptuous, ordinary people, singers, writers, directors, industrialists, sportsmen, failed promises or crushed careers, lost children, desperate mothers.

Thus, little by little, my very personal toolbox became more articulate, varied and rich in resources.

The strangest room? A lawn!

I was on duty; the atmosphere was calm. Everyone is asleep. Or almost everyone.

It starts when a young patient decides to leave in the middle of the night, without any warning or asking permission. This acute emergency is also delicate to handle. He is one of the "professor's" patients. He is agitated, at risk, and must be found as soon as possible. A quick decision: I consult the head nurse and leave the clinic to go and look for him. Two nurses accompany me. As I imagined, the fugitive has taken refuge in a nearby golf clubhouse. Meeting, negotiations, more or less consensual sedative therapy. Everything OK? Not even close! In a fraction of a second, the young man jumps to his feet, opens the French window onto the lawn and starts running across *the fairways* of the golf course, pursued by the improvised medical team. Fortunately, it was a hilly course, the medication was starting to work, and the long night was taking its toll, and the patient was "retrieved" and taken back to the clinic.

It is not the first or last time that the room has been transformed into a mobile intervention unit.

It is the fate and fortune of young doctors. It is called a home visit.

For therapies, check-ups, intravenous treatments, consultations, and all kinds of emergencies.

Misery and degradation, waiting behind doors that will never open, rejection, insults, threats, humiliation. Despondency, a lot of it, accompanied by a sense of powerlessness. Or, sometimes, omnipotence. Which, in the end, is the same thing.

Like that time I found myself in a beautiful house in an exclusive neighbourhood of Milan: as I walked down the corridor to reach the bedroom of my patient, the only son of the owners of the house, I recognised some Fontana (unframed, of course) among other paintings of equal value, and I became breathless when the mother appeared, one of the most beautiful women I have ever met.

Getting paid for my visits took time and patience. My witty analyst suggested that I propose that I receive one of the paintings (even without a frame) as payment for my professional services.

These, of course, remained where they were, while the payments arrived after multiple and prolonged bouts of amnesia. It was a good lesson in humility. Entering other people's rooms makes you feel powerful, important, respected, even feared, and I, at that time, a young novice, went from euphoria (at having been chosen by an important family) to a sense of deep frustration, since not being paid coincided with a lack of recognition. In my profession, it is easy to get caught up in dangerous feelings of arrogance and omniscience. Experiencing the opposite – a state of fragility – guarantees a reset and repositions the centre of gravity of our therapeutic function where it rightfully belongs.

The room is also a "safe" place for a therapist, whether young or old.

Psychoanalysts of my generation were given strict rules of conduct in case we ever happened to meet patients outside the office, entirely by chance, of course.

So, there is no shortage of tragicomic anecdotes about colleagues who avoided leaving the house, fleeing from one pavement to another, experiencing spatial and temporal disorientation, episodes of prosopagnosia, suddenly leaving theatres or cinemas (even a front row seat at La Scala), and behaviour on the brink of rudeness. In short, it shouldn't have happened. And yet we meet a patient. Cycling in the city, in a small town at a Swiss border crossing, queuing for a ski lift, on an intercontinental flight, in a London museum while holding your granddaughter, at a dessert buffet at the end of a wedding. Reminding us that life continues to flow outside and beyond our studios. In these cases – we must remember – we are no longer the masters of the room, because we are no longer in those safe boundaries, the outside world belongs to everyone, first and foremost the patient that we may meet, who may not want to greet us, nor give any clue to others that may be with them that they know us. In short, they decide.

Then the rooms, like humans, age, become defined, are entrusted, assigned with a nameplate, first and last name. Finally, personalised with paintings, posters, photos and memories.

"Mine."

I have changed four private practices so far, but my fondest, most deeply-rooted memories always go back to the very first one, that will remain with me forever. And I would not want to lose it for anything in the world. My parents' generosity and foresight allowed me to have it. A home/practice. While waiting for it to be ready, an equally generous and trusting colleague sent me my first official patient. I couldn't keep her waiting; she wasn't well, and she might have gone to see someone else. So, in no time at all, I set up a decent room with some sparse furniture, and the table in particular, which I still use today. The only thing missing was the "waiting room", who knows what for, that I set up in the corridor/entrance room.

I had fallen in love with a Vienna straw bench by Lyda Levi. It was rather unusual, and required a long production time, that didn't meet my deadline or the urgent need of the patient. Thanks to a good deal of determined persuasion, I managed to get it delivered on a Monday morning. My helpful mother had guaranteed her presence at that time to pick it up. I was going to see the new patient that same afternoon. Everything seemed ready. Unfortunately, the coveted – indispensable? – bench smelled like fresh paint, like a newly sanded parquet floor. I am still fond of that bench today, but I continue to hold it responsible, and it suits me, for the immediate interruption or failure to start my first therapy. I think I smelled a little too new myself!

I have always shared my office with the same colleague; we have collaborated both personally and professionally for almost 40 years. We made sacrifices and took turns using the first office, the one with the bench which was only one room. But when, a few years later, we had the opportunity to change offices, I must confess with a bit of embarrassment that I demanded that there should also be two waiting rooms in addition to the two rooms, which we now needed. This is a good opportunity to admit to her that I was really exaggerating, since she was, after all, both the victim and accomplice of my arrogance.

It was then that the much coveted and feared couch made its entrance into the room. I had carefully chosen the version, black, *total black*. There could be no doubt about the model, I had wanted it all my life. Both of my analysts, personal and training, obviously had this same Le Corbusier's chaise longue. Even the room seemed happy, more at ease, and in order, having a more precisely defined identity.

The problem was considering it the centrepiece, the very soul of the place, the one on which all patients, sooner or later, would have to lie down.

M-A-N-D-A-T-O-R-Y

Then things change. The same couch is still there. But its function has changed: anyone can use it or not use it at all, as they choose, in their own time and in their own way. Some people, a few, start from the beginning, some after a while, some intermittently, some just to rest or see what it feels like, some while continuing to maintain eye contact, some with one foot on the floor, some never.

In complete, total freedom.

Once they become patients, people do not always serenely accept changes in the room. Some come to try to change, but they need secure, stable references. Somehow, they resemble children in this. Sometimes they don't even see what the room looks like.

After weeks, months or years, much to their surprise, they discover the existence of a plant that is almost 3 metres tall. Or a certain painting, a piece of furniture. Others, on the other hand, analyse it as if they possessed a scanner instead of eyes. Some rejoice in the change, especially if it is associated with a pleasant or familiar memory ("How nice, it's on the street where my old nursery school was!"), while the novelty causes others to suffer.

This is why, despite the inevitable changes, it is important that the room retains its identity. It remains itself. This is what gives the therapist true security, the freedom to experiment beyond rigid, pre-established scripts.

I remember a young patient admitted to a clinic in Milan where I was working at the time. Rosalia oscillated between severe depression and delusional, threatening and cosmic ideas. Both conditions always led to the same the result: she never improved and also never washed. She was as beautiful as a Madonna by Antonello da Messina but started to smell worse and worse. Entering her room for consultations was risky. And bringing her to the office for interviews kept it out of use for a few hours. In the summer, it was easier, as the windows could be thrown open. In winter, the issue was more complex.

One day, at the end of my shift, I said to her sadly, as I opened the French window as wide as possible: "Rosalia, if today you won't wash yourself, I swear that tomorrow I'll bring you the musical ball that my daughter uses in the bath and see if that makes it easier for you!" Well, I would never have believed what ensued. Somehow, the sense of paternal attention to her body – compensating for a deep sense of abandonment by her own father – was enough for Rosalia to show up for the interview the next day washed, perfumed and with her long raven-black hair loose on her shoulders.

Creativity is, in fact, sometimes necessary in therapy. And on this note, I am reminded of Arianna, a confused and weary young woman, stuck in an *impasse* that prevented her from finding her place in the world and making her own choices. Her family wanted a future for her that was at odds with her artistic and contemplative nature. She liked acting and dancing, but she was afraid she wouldn't be able to do it, that she wasn't capable. It wasn't easy for her to attend the sessions. She feared the normative and controlling aspects, the possibility of being bent to her family's wishes.

One day she entered the studio dressed as a mime, like Marcel Marceau, and asked if she could stage a *play*. She began to unravel a ball of red thread, weaving countless patterns connecting all the objects in the room in a sort of net that also included me. She danced between the threads, above and below, without even touching them. She ended the intense performance with a sort of Argentine tango casque, throwing banknotes into the air that corresponded exactly to the cost of a session. She received enthusiastic applause even before words and interpretations. This was the confirmation that she needed to feel that during therapy she could truly explore any aspect of her hopes and dreams without limits. And thus, free to experiment and test her skills and passions, she finally could choose without having to oppose.

And then there were also sessions standing up, walking around, coming and going and running away, and sometimes some people even lay on the floor, we swapped places between the patient's chair and my armchair, a black and somewhat imposing Stokke – a throne, as a teenager once said. It could have certainly seemed strange, even bizarre, if someone had a glimpse of us working in reversed positions. I think it helped the patient as much as it helped me.

In the room, I found myself "imitating" the posture and voice or tone of my interlocutors. It sounds like a story of mockery. For many, it was a chance to be seen and recognised.

Tommaso Senise, one of my teachers, taught me that apart from a couple of things that should never be done – everyone should know what – anything can be done in therapy, if you know why you are doing it.

So new objects entered the room: photographs, games, balls, films, musical instruments, computers, video games.

Not just in stories, but as concrete objects. Even various breeds of dogs. The practice is *pet friendly*, as animals also represent internal aspects of the people who bring them. Just like the friend that a young patient brought into the room with her one day. She wanted to convince her to start psychotherapy and had decided that the best way would be to let her attend a live session. So much for confidentiality.

What is the room, my room, like now?

After a small move to another floor, it is not very different from how it has always been, at least in my mind.

It is the place where I spend and have spent most of my life. That's also why, out of care and respect for myself and for those who enter it, I like to keep it tidy and clean. Ideally, I would like it to always smell nice, which is important, so I have installed an air purifier. There used to be a warm-toned Persian rug, but now there is a more practical floor covering in a light colour. Different images hang on the walls. Diplomas, mementos, an exhibition poster of Freud drawn by Valerio Adami, a much-loved painter, photos of landscapes and people. A watercolour found under my parents' bed – *Encounter* – depicts two indistinct figures approaching each other.

A painting that I really adore is in one corner; unfortunately, it's a bit hidden. It depicts the boundary between inside and outside, a space, perhaps. A room, which you can enter or leave. It was done by an artist I admire, Davide Pizzigoni, a dear friend. In another corner, there is a new green plant. The first one had grown relentlessly to the ceiling for 35 years. My connection with nature inside the room was a source of pride. Nina Coltart – the great British psychoanalyst who helped us think the unthinkable – always reminded us that every therapist should own and cultivate a garden. There is a plaster bas-relief, *La Gradiva*, almost hidden behind the plant. This is a reproduction of the copy purchased by Freud in 1906 at the Vatican

Museums. It was donated by Cesare Musatti to Milanese psychoanalysts in the 1960s, is a symbol of belonging, and has been now replicated for everyone. Then there are a few books and magazines, neatly arranged in the bookcase, the chairs are comfortable, the curtains gently protect the room yet leave us a glimpse of the city, the walls have been donned with colours to convey tranquillity. All these details are my way of welcoming people. Treatment begins there too.

And finally, there are many small objects, gifts and mementos, each with a story, that watch me from the metal shelves and dark wood of the desk. Only I am keenly aware of their value.

Here, time flows at its own pace.

Sometimes it seems to slow down or expand, as if silently indulging in the mood of my patients, the flow of their words, sometimes torrential, sometimes reticent. It is a pleasant feeling, even if sometimes managing the minutes that pass, hinting towards the end and closing a session is not simple. After all, this is also part of my job: to stay on course, to gently guide the flow of thoughts, and discretely distribute the pauses.

Perhaps it is because I like being here and I am not tired of it yet.

The only thing that bothers me about this room is having to sit still for so long. Moving around and using my body has always been important to me. So, when I can, I get up, stretch my legs a little, and do some conscious movements. And I allow myself to use my room too. The ergonomic reclining chair, sometimes even the couch also grants me welcoming minutes of relaxation, rest and reflection. Then the sound of the intercom, the buzzing of the doorbell, an alarm on my phone brings me back to my senses and the sense of the room, the reason for having created it, for living in it.

In this book, my present room, and all my past rooms, have been opened. And they have revealed that each new patient is an encounter, an unknown world to discover, or rediscover, together. From here on, the inhabitants, more or less temporary, will speak up and will tell their stories. My patients and myself will talk about what can happen in this place and how it can be seen by people who enter it for the first time.

2 Premises, Expectations, Encounters

Psychoanalysts are not neutral static entities to fill up. They are people nourished by the encounters, who must treat other people, but also treat themselves.

The patient expects the psychoanalyst not to have overly strong tones or smells, to create a welcoming space. At the same time, this reassuring opacity must hint at depth.

The patient trusts, and the psychoanalyst trusts too, albeit in a different way. How, exactly?

In the room, where it is impossible to simulate another profession, psychoanalysts have long "hidden" behind the issue of neutrality, trying to resolve it skilfully, partly through anonymity (sitting behind a couch also helps) and partly through mystery. This is necessary to some extent. No one goes to a therapist to find out what they are like or what kind of life they lead, but to be listened to, understood, even revealed, in part or in whole. Themselves, not the therapist.

However, if, as is evident, there are two or more people in the room, at least one of them is the analyst. And we must begin to deal with this other inhabitant. He must enter the scene and at this point, begin to describe, beyond the concrete aspects of the place and the patient's world, something more about what happens in his – in my – world.

Every day, at every possible hour, somewhere, someone is getting ready to come to me. Facing long journeys, rush-hour traffic, escaping from the office, daily worries, last-minute setbacks, sudden second thoughts. Some with great enthusiasm, others with reluctance. Even following precise rituals. Calmly. Or in a hurry.

"What should I wear? Smart, casual or not even think about it? And my hair, my make-up. How?"

I'm on this side too. "How do I look, what do I do, how do I prepare for the meeting?"

It's funny, even romantic, to think that we are preparing for the same event, albeit from such different perspectives and in such different roles but doing more or less the same things. At the end of the day, we're not so different.

DOI: 10.4324/9781003759034-2

Let's start at the beginning of the day.

I like early mornings, their solitude, that sense of isolation and tranquillity that the early hours convey.

A glance out of the window, life getting underway, the sky, the weather, the forecast, the changing light depending on the season. Small rituals, small reassuring and familiar routines. Like checking emails, glimpsing at the news, some gentle grooming for the body and soul. A nice and necessary breakfast.

A review of the agenda.

I usually know who is coming and when, the sequence is clearly imprinted in my mind.

Every day and every moment have its protagonists. Then we have the "new guests", the first visits, the requests. New emotions.

Not all days are the same, nor are people. I know full well that there are peaceful, even pleasant days and encounters, and others that are less so. There are patients who provoke negative emotions in us, beyond any stereotype or code of silence. It is only if we can accept and recognise what we feel and sense that we can learn to manage it, without being overwhelmed and conditioned by it.

The morning rituals including preparing the room and the atmosphere require time and attention. Lights, intercoms, doorbells, viewers and fans, air conditioning in summer, heaters in winter. Everything must be ready. Music and candies for the waiting room. A sort of antechamber, preparing patients for the actual room. Some people like to spend time there before the session, some sleep there, some stand, some would like to avoid it and get straight to the point. For many, it is like a decompression chamber (perhaps spending time there regularly is a substantial part of the treatment). For me it is an almost sacred, protected place. I have always tried to take care of this space. Muffled, soundproofed, discreetly lit, separate but connected. Truly delicate. Organised to avoid inappropriate and unwelcome encounters. To be defended as much as, if not more than, privacy regulations. Even though this is not always possible, despite our best efforts.

Like that time when, accompanying a patient to the door, we met the next one who was coming in. The two looked at each other for a moment, then smiled and hugged each other warmly. They were two dear friends, neither of whom knew that the other was in therapy, let alone with the same therapist. Or another occasion when I realised from two successive rings of the intercom that, between rescheduling and rearranging appointments, I had apparently given two different people appointments at the same time. I opened the door to the waiting room, ready to offer my apologies, when I saw the two patients sitting on the same sofa, chatting amiably. They were colleagues who hadn't seen each other for some time, and as they talked, they discovered unexpected similarities. Almost a friendship. In both cases, I felt like a stranger, practically almost out of place. I remained observing the scene. I thought that perhaps they would have preferred to be left alone to continue their conversation.

My arrival in the room, along with my interlocutors, is both the last and first act of a process that began a long, long time ago. The end of the process of getting there; the start of the road ahead. For me, it began with my decision to do this job and shut myself away for countless hours of my life within these four walls.

Right from the first contact, whether it is a fortunate coincidence between the phone call and my availability to answer, a message on the answering machine (and the time to call back), an email explaining and motivating the request, a text message or a WhatsApp message, that is the very moment that gives birth to our first meeting, that amazing opportunity, always suspended between surprise and the unknown.

To facilitate this, clear and detailed directions are needed to reach the building, enter the office and take a seat in the waiting room. Even though there is always someone who misses the instructions, gets the street number wrong, follows a satnav that takes them to the right address but in a small village in the hinterland, or confuses the day and time.

The magic of waiting begins to unfold in that space. Who is looking for me? Who will arrive? Will they be young, adult, mature, elderly? A beautiful person, or ugly, or indifferent? Will I like them? Will they like me? Will I be able to help them? Will I know how to help them? What will become of us?

These are the moments before the meeting, my own private mental waiting room where emotions and thoughts race through my mind. If my future interlocutors spend their time in the gardens near the studio or by the door of the building, waiting for the right moment to ring the bell? I am inside the room also grinding away at the anticipation of what will happen and when it will happen, between early arrivals (*how anxious…*), punctuality (*how precise…*) and delays (*where could they be… will he ever arrive?)*, ghosts and *desaparecidos (*often without warning or justification for their absence).

Because it is quite easy to make an appointment, more or less difficult to keep it, but very easy to disregard or cancel it, especially at the last minute, with a simple tap on the keyboard of your mobile phone or computer. Keeping the acquired right to the reserved space but exercising total freedom to do without it without hesitation or penalty, new inhabitants of an illusory Olympus of the gods of "everything is permitted". A rather popular Olympus, moreover.

The patient's (or customer's, if you will) life is certainly a hard one, but the life of those who must wait is not any easier, always powerless in the face of others' decisions.

Waiting, in fact.

Some fill waiting with nothing, perhaps the "healthiest" choice; others, however, fill it with various forms and methods.

It used to be easier to remain anonymous; people would introduce themselves with their story. Sometimes with a more or less well-known name and surname, a sort of pre-introduction, which was unavoidable. Now, the immense database of the web and social media speak extensively about us and them, whether we want it (often) or not.

We can lose so much surprise and amazement in this way. How many fantasies and expectations we create within ourselves with our somewhat futile attempts to anticipate and predict what will happen. This temptation is difficult to avoid in a digital world that always tells stories about us, even if we don't want it to and try to avoid it. Just think of the social media profiles that offer us photos or images of people we will meet – all they need to do is write a message or an email. It's no big deal, it happens to me too, you just need to know how to use it properly and wisely. Like everything else.

Here we are.

With a slight uneasiness mixed with physiological curiosity, I walk down the short, sometimes interminable, sometimes very short corridor that separates my room from the waiting room. In those moments, when I am more aware, my thoughts turn to *La stanza del figlio* [*The Son's Room*], the film in which Nanni Moretti, in the role of psychoanalyst Giovanni Sermonti, walks down the corridor separating his office from his home. Thoughtful, still immersed in the atmosphere after the appointments with his patients, he walks and, with every step, taps his hand on the wall. Every day, several times a day, I also cross that space back and forth and measure it with my steps and with my hands tapping softly on the walls as if to test them, perhaps to greet them.

Now I am at the door of the waiting room, the wait is over, I open it, look inside and finally see (meeting and getting to know each other will come later, hopefully) the person who will spend at least the next 45 minutes with me. A quick but cordial introduction. I have my ritual – exchanging first and last names, making eye contact and shaking hands – but everyone has their own, which must be respected, understood and considered. You may love or hate physical contact, looking people in the face, sideways or down. Those few moments already say a lot about us. I make a mental note of them, smile and extend my arm with my hand open, followed by an invitation to head towards the room down the corridor. They are in front; I stay behind. A small procession that everyone does as they see fit, some almost running, others with careful caution. And I adapt, a tortoise with the tortoises, a hare with the hares. A good preview of what our meeting and subsequent journey will be like, travelled at the pace and speed decided by our interlocutors.

Finally, we reach the room – what a tiring and long introduction – the meeting really begins.

For example, like this.

When I restarted sessions in September after summer holidays, Cecilia asked me for an appointment. From our exchanges – emails, text messages and minutes – aimed at laboriously finding a slot, I had formulated the idea that she was a psychologist enrolled in a school of psychotherapy. I had in mind that after the first interview, I could refer her to a colleague if necessary. On the day of our first meeting, shortly after opening both the front door and entrance door for her, the intercom suddenly rings again, signalling the arrival of another patient, and I realise that I have given her the wrong time, 45 minutes early. I am bitter and sorry. It is not the first time this has happened, and I blame my own foolishness. I am also a little agitated by the mistake, so I try to calm myself with a few deep breaths and go to let her know. I am greeted by a smiling, pleasant face. We introduce ourselves; I apologise for the mistake and ask her if she can come back when I am free. She seems to have been expecting this. Evidently, the sound of the intercom had put her on alert.

"No problem!" she says, calmly heading for the exit.

"Thank you, I'll explain what happened later..."

She returns punctually, we meet again, I apologise once more, I explain the reasons, she says it's not necessary, I do it anyway (incorrect reading of the timeline on the electronic diary), she appreciates it. She makes no mention of the incident.

She begins to talk about why she is there; a decision made in the summer after much deliberation. She knows nothing about analysis and psychotherapy but asks to begin a course of treatment to get to know herself and feel better about herself, her husband and her baby daughter. It sounds like the kind of request psychoanalysts used to receive in the mid-twentieth century. She is a very pleasant person who works in healthcare. This also surprises me. Contrary to my prejudices, I imagine that I could take her on for analysis. I become more involved. I think it is necessary to ask her to become more involved too. I try to test her willingness/ability to work on herself. So, halfway through the interview, I decide to return to the initial misunderstanding, asking her how she felt about my mistake.

"Nothing, I went shopping for tonight, since we invited some friends over for drinks. I told my husband and he was happy!"

"Good, this highlights your ability to adapt and turn problems into opportunities. However, you talked about doing... let's try to go back and try to get in touch with what you felt?"

"That you were clear, explicit, that you seemed to be strong, confident... authoritative."

"OK, now we've accessed your thoughts, what you thought... but... what did you feel?"

"Empathy... it happens, it has happened to me with my patients, I consoled myself... it can happen..."

"OK... we're in touch, so... and nothing else? ... no negative feelings... only positive emotions and thoughts...?"

"Yes!"

"What if you tried to consider what your patients feel or have felt on those occasions?"

"Generally, they understand... we apologise... we are kind. My colleague and friend and I often think that patients recognise that we are young, pretty and courteous... they tell us so directly. And sometimes we ask ourselves: will we always be like this? Or will we also become unpleasant, aloof and unhelpful over time? As we often see in our older colleagues..."

"Are you talking about me too?" We smile together.

A good meeting, no doubt about it. Is it always like this?

I would like to say yes, to tell stories of smooth sailing, magical encounters, immediate and easy understanding, of journeys that begin quickly and end harmoniously, but that would be a poor imitation of a Walt Disney film or a scene from *Pollyanna*. Fortunately, there are encounters like the one I have just described, but my room is often the witness and guardian of much more complicated and controversial moments, in which understanding each other and truly understanding what is happening in the other person is a real challenge.

"What's happening to you? Can I help you?"

This is the question that crosses my mind every time I meet a new person. Patients no longer come to us with the absolute conviction that they wanted to begin analysis with complete trust and openness. In the middle of the last century, psychoanalysis was the only psychological therapy available and operated as a monopoly. As we well know, if there is no competition, there is no evolution, no improvement, just resting on one's laurels.

Over the last 40 years, other psychological therapies have been developed that have helped people, have been validated through empirical research, and seek to offer comprehensive and articulated responses to psychological needs and suffering. Comparing different techniques and models can stimulate, enrich and enhance our discipline, making us better at what we do, without fear of rivalry.

Nowadays, when a person arrives, notwithstanding they are suffering and in need, they come equipped with their own baggage of information and knowledge (including prejudices, of course) that become an integral part of the encounter and the response to their request. We are obliged to engage in dialogue and negotiation.

The most attentive psychoanalysts now ask themselves: "Which therapy for which patient?"

I totally agree with this and try to integrate this philosophy in every moment of my work.

I hope that sooner or later we will reach a situation in which a clinician acts according to this sequence: he meets a person, tries to understand his problem and recommends the most suitable psychological therapy, even if he is not the one who practises it.

Meanwhile, the interview with Cecilia has ended, we have decided to meet again, we are giving ourselves time to understand each other and decide what to do with our meeting and our time.

For now, we have made a start.

Anita – Monday, 7.45 a.m.

I've made up my mind. I can't take it anymore. I have no strength, no courage, can't even muster up smile. No more will. I don't know if they sell it at the supermarket or the chemists. Mine has run out.

I look for a name, I ask around, I find out information, I do my research on the internet.

I have a name, a surname and a telephone number, even an email address.

It takes me a while to dial the number. For some people, the post-it note with the reminder stays on the fridge for days, months, even years, forgotten on the desk, lost in a wallet. It would be easy to retrieve it. If I were healthy. Instead, I get paranoid.

It's just like teenagers in love who want to make their first phone call: panic. Because as soon as someone on the other end answers, it's done: you're already naked, you've exposed yourself and there's no turning back. In the end, desperation wins out.

I call, hoping that the doctor will answer and give me an appointment for the same day, even now would be fine, right away. Instead, I get the answering machine.

The recorded voice says to leave a name and telephone number, and you will be contacted as soon as possible. It's even polite, but nothing. I freeze. I hang up. Panic, again. I call back.

Then, finally, with the most decent voice I can muster, I leave my message, hang up and from that moment on I can't stop looking at my mobile phone. I go to the bathroom with my mobile phone, I charge it as soon as I can, any other calls are just a nuisance, I want the line free.

Finally, the doctor calls. The appointment is for the following week.

I thank him, hang up and say to myself, OK, let's hope we make it to next week.

From that moment on, the *countdown* begins, objectively heading towards the only hope I have left.

When the fateful day arrives, I am there half an hour early. I smoke a thousand cigarettes in front of the intercom. I take a walk, come back, there is still plenty of time, another thousand cigarettes. Only when my desperate anticipation begins to take on the characteristics of polite anticipation – about ten minutes for me – do I ring the intercom. The door opens with a click.

I climb the steps; the front door is on the left. I ring the bell, another click.

I enter. At least I passed the practical intelligence test. Here I am in the hall.

There is a tiny bench on the right. Am I supposed to sit there? It's so small! What if it breaks? Maybe it's another test. In fact, there is another door on the left. Next to it, on the wall, I see a sign.

"Waiting room. Come in." I obey.

I open the glass door – it's heavy – I throw myself inside, and it closes behind me.

I sit down, glance at the magazines, the paintings, the carpet, hear the music in the background, admire the giant plant, eye the candies, but don't dare go near them, take a deep breath and wait.

Alessandra – Monday, 8.45 a.m.

Even the unconscious has an antechamber. At least, mine does.

It is a waiting room with a door that closes by itself. You open it, enter and choose where to sit.

There are two places, on a two-seater sofa on the right, soft, warm and comfortable.

Three other places on a Vienna straw sofa, a little more austere.

And three single seats: two right in front of the door, one to the side. They are comfortable, but metallic, cold.

I wonder why there are so many options.

Perhaps it means that there is a place for each of us. For our shapes, needs and habits.

The first time, still looking for the right seat for me, I hear music in the background. I later realised that it was a compilation playing on a loop. To me, it seems perfect every time. Perhaps I am lucky in this respect, at least.

Other people may not like it. It is not easy to please everyone.

Offering many options may also suggest something about those who chose them. There is no doubt that I am the object of the study, but if you have a little free time, you can also get an idea of who the doctor is from the chairs and music.

There is a plant at the back, in front of the window, it's a kentia, which provides the room stunning and comforting beauty.

There are photos on the walls: lighthouses in the sea on the left wall, mountain peaks on the right wall and, on the wall by the door, there is the Dr Jekyll of humanity, Tibet or Nepal, I don't know, but it is a civilisation that certainly does not think about cosmetic surgery.

I don't think they were placed there randomly; nothing seems random. Like in a puzzle magazine, when you think you've deciphered the arcane meaning, right or wrong, you feel clever and proud.

No other voices can be heard.

Everything is muffled, soundproofed. You are there, you must stay there, you stay there. Protected, and held.

It's a nice feeling.

The highlight of the waiting room is the basket full of candies.

The liquorice ones are the best in the world, and that's an objective fact.

In my opinion, the first thing people do when they enter is to rummage through the little basket, discard the *jellies*, hesitate over the *mou*, identify their prey and pop it into their mouth. Some, with childish nostalgia, choose the *Galatine*.

There you go. It's the taste of the antechamber of my unconscious. Let's go back to choosing where to sit.

I bet that every patient has said to themselves at least once: "Blimey, choosing where to sit could mean something, but I can't imagine what, although I'm sure the doctor will surely decipher it, and so… If I sit with my back to the door, it could mean that I'm trying to hide, and that's not good. If I sit facing the door, I might reveal an aggressive, defensive attitude, so not that either. The sofa, on the other hand, could be interpreted as a relaxed state of mind, which I don't have. So, what then?"

The reasoning lasts ten seconds at most, which is enough to realise that it's all nonsense. Sit down and *fuck off*, you're there to try to figure out what even you don't know about yourself, it's not a chair that's going to change your life.

Later, I would have chosen the sofa and looked at the photographs of the lighthouses on the wall. But the first few times, I would sit next to the door. Ready to run away? I know very little about myself.

I really struggle to describe myself. That's why I'm here. What could I say? That I'm small, compact, curvy. Pretty. That's for sure. A pretty face, a bright white smile on an olive complexion. All I need is a mole, a third eye on my forehead, and there you have an Indian woman. I am truly a stranger in my own country.

I sit and look at the carpet.

This carpet knows how to tell its story.

I begin to fantasise. I like to invent stories. To imagine. It's my job, it comes easily to me.

Originally it was a precious carpet, it was adopted and brought into a home where it remained for years. Then, one terrible day, someone tripped and spilled a dark liquid – tea or coffee – on it. The stain clearly shows that everything possible was done to remove it, but unfortunately, it didn't work. Carpets with these stories, just like sofas, usually go from homes to offices. Too beautiful to throw away, too stained to leave on display. I love that carpet. It may seem strange, but I really love it. Perhaps because we are both imperfect, and in the same way I would like to be recovered, even recycled would be fine.

Time slows down in the antechamber of the unconscious.

You try to gather your thoughts and remember everything you had planned to say to the doctor in the previous days, and you can't wait for that door to open. You can't, because you can't, but along with the fuss about where to sit, I bet that every patient, at least once, has had to curb the instinct to throw their arms around his neck and cry their heart out. It's happened to me loads of times, every time I've come back from holiday. The joy of seeing your doctor again is overwhelming. You wag your tail like a little dog from the morning onwards, and when he opens the door and you find yourself in front of him, what the fuck, do you only shake his hand? At the very least, you hug him and say, always addressing him formally and with your best smile: "You bastard, I missed you so much!" But you don't do that.

Always shake hands, no matter what.

And that's what I do, thinking that he knows how I feel.

Unfortunately, after a few months, the Master of the World made his appearance in "my" waiting room. In his forties, a light brown-haired Big Jim, with light eyes, light trousers, light-framed glasses and an even lighter rudeness mixed with aggression.

The waiting room should be a private place. It is the place where you disconnect from the outside world and focus on your inner self. You don't joke around there. You don't chat. And if there is another person, sometimes even more than one, you greet them, but no small talk. If you are in there, at least as far as I'm concerned, it means that you have crossed over to the other side, to the world of "others" – you have left the "normal" people behind. It means that you have experienced a reality that most people will never even fathom and that your point of view has inevitably changed, forever.

And so, you demand respect and seriousness.

Instead, "the arsehole", while he threw the door open as if there were a fire, turns on the light, which goes from dim to blinding. He stocks up on what are objectively the best liquorice candies in the world, sometimes mumbles a greeting, often not. As soon as he sits down, always facing the door, he receives a phone call, clearly with the ring tone on full volume, and he starts talking at full volume. I wonder why he always arrives so early, disturbing my magical moment.

I'm going to kill him. It's the only thing that calmly comes to mind, as if it were the only possible solution to a tedious problem that I've already had the opportunity to evaluate.

Yes, yes. I'll kill him.

The bastard brings you back to the outside world. That's what makes you furious.

He's not doing what everyone should be doing, and his behaviour is preventing you from doing what you need to do. Because patients have responsibilities too, for fuck's sake. And so, while he talks loudly, munching noisily on his candy, I glare at him. Months have passed since he first appeared, and now we're at loggerheads. I always arrive before him. One day, after he didn't even say hello to me twice in a row, I looked him straight in the eye and said:

H-E-L-L-O-!

I think I was quite clear and effective because he always says hello to me now.

He knows I hate him, but he doesn't care.

What he doesn't know is that one day he'll stop yelling on the phone because I'll find the strength to kill him.

And what he doesn't know, above all, is that he's dealing with someone who is his exact opposite.

I know he's the Master of the World, but he doesn't know that I am the Non-Existent.

I know that his obnoxious attitude stems from an experience in which you either impose yourself or succumb. He chose the former. I chose the latter.

And here we are, in the same room. It doesn't surprise me at all. Neither of us should have had to live through that situation, that's all. We weren't protected, and each of us did what we did to be able to cope: we tried things out.

All things considered, I may not kill him after all.

The door to the waiting room has a frosted glass panel.

When a patient leaves the doctor's room, you catch a glimpse of their shadow and realise that your turn is coming.

Your 45 minutes.

Shortly afterwards, more or less on time, the door opens for me, my doctor appears in the doorway, and his reassuring smile appears with him.

"Good morning, Alessandra."

"Good morning, Doctor."

We shake hands and go in, ready to begin our journey.

Simona – Monday, 9.45 a.m.

A few signals vaguely announce his presence. Noises, lights coming on in the anteroom and doors opening and closing and then Doc suddenly appears in the doorway of the waiting room.

He now crosses the same threshold I crossed earlier.

The fact that he comes to get me is wonderful! No secretaries or formalities.

He has a gentle air, is dressed elegantly but not ostentatiously, and wears comfortable English lace-up shoes: he is a psychiatrist and is ready for anything. Even me.

He gives me a questioning but confident look, saying my first and last name. He extends his hand and tells me his first and last name.

Perhaps that may be just enough to feel recognised.

After all, we are all just a first name and a surname. He invites me to follow him.

The journey is short, but it can seem endless. Awkwardness. "Doctor," I wonder to myself, "do you peek at your patients during those few metres? At what your patients are like?"

I look at everything.

"And what do you think of their shoes?" For me, they are fundamental.

I enter the office and feel, even before speaking, that I would like to pitch a nice camping tent and stay there for at least a month straight.

I sit down in the chair opposite him. We start talking.

I would like to tell him a million things, but I have already come up with the most concise and meaningful formula.

"I think I have a brain tumour, or something like that. Frankly, I can no longer bear the pain I feel or the voices I hear. My brain is literally boiling. The only thing I've really wanted for some time now is to die. The voices aren't someone else's, they're just my thoughts overlapping, you know like when an equalizer breaks in a piece of music. And then, really, I don't feel understood by anyone, but who can understand something like that? That's why I want to kill myself. There's no turning back from here. Or is there?"

He's not a magician, even though I wish he were, he made me talk, he asked me questions, and from time to time he waited, as if to invite me to continue.

He's not a magician, as I said, and the answer came in the end.

"The symptoms you've described have nothing to do with a brain tumour or any other incurable disease, if anything, they're related with an illness that is completely treatable – depression. If you agree, we can embark on a journey together. Are you willing to take medication? Good, so take this medicine I'm prescribing, and you should start to feel better after a couple of weeks, certainly after four, but believe me, you can make it: there is no need to commit suicide."

Giving up on your plans is not easy, especially when they seem to solve all your problems.

I had done everything to keep them and make them happen. Tenaciously, insistently. And the Doc, with his proposal, was screwing me over.

We made an appointment for the following week, he gave me the prescription for the medication, showed me to the door, then another handshake and a smile.

"See you on Monday?"

"See you on Monday," I replied. And I smiled too.

This meant that I would not commit suicide until the following week.

I turned around, ran down the steps and, once outside the front door, leaned my whole body against the wall. My heart was racing and in a second, I burst into tears. I was relieved that I didn't have a brain tumour but scared because I was still suffering from a severe depression.

And I had a sense of bewilderment because my mother had always suffered from depression but had never sought treatment.

I cried, feeling monstrously fragile, but relieved.

I finally knew that it wasn't my fault, it wasn't my fault, the doctor had been very clear.

"The feelings and emotions you experience are caused by the illness, not you. Now we are treating the illness, so the symptoms will gradually disappear."

It didn't seem possible, but it was true.

I tried to pull myself together, dried my tears, clutched the prescription in my hand and went straight to the chemist's. They knew me, of course, it was close to home, and I had lived there for years. I waited until all the customers had left and only then did I hand the prescription to the chemist.

He read the name of the medicine, and I thought I saw a flash of surprise in his eyes, but his voice was warm and affectionate: "Hey, what's going on?"

I didn't answer, I just started crying again. So, he disappeared into the back and came back with the medicine.

"Don't worry, please! Everything will be fine, you'll see."

I nodded and, without saying a word, left with a small bag.

The medicine that would save my life, together with the Doc and other key people.

3 Adolescence

Throughout my professional life I have dedicated a very particular attention to my work with adolescents. I take care of them. I feel comfortable with them, a kind of comfort zone.

Where does this feeling come from? How did it start?

Every psychoanalyst should understand his choices are largely dictated by distant and personal events. So, the reason that led me to work with young people is part of my history, it has roots in the boy and son I was, and in the way I went through that phase of life.

As the eldest child and a model student – and therefore not particularly popular with my peers – when I entered adolescence, I had to deal with a series of house moves, environmental changes and school transfers that could be comparable to micro-emigrations. I found myself being tossed about, forced to frequently change peer groups and always making new acquaintances and points of reference. I remember long afternoons spent on a basketball court in a youth religious club, playing around on my own with a ball. Playing sports saved me a little, even though it isolated me. I was shy and inhibited. This alienating feeling stayed with me for a long time, like a mark or an identity. I found my usual friends and acquaintances only during the summer – I called myself *a summer boy* – in the holiday resort, which fortunately never changed. Every year, September was synonymous with the end of my illusion of a normal life. Obviously, I blamed my parents for all this. In my eyes, they were responsible for the upheavals in my life, the end of my summer dreams, the friends I lost, the girls I had to say goodbye to with the vein hope of finding them unchanged the following summer.

At home, I was impatient and unbearable. I encountered the first stirrings and echoes of 1968, still *in its infancy.* Politics was a way to get out on the streets and discover the world. I didn't understand anything about right and left, fascism and communism; my head was really confused. I drew random symbols on the military backpack I bought at the Fiera di Sinigaglia, Milan's most beloved flea market. But I believe that a certain oratorical ease originated during this time of groups, assemblies, demonstrations, slogans and books, where I created my small vital niche, helping to melt my shyness and fuel my pleasure in speaking in public and being listened to. A few good human

DOI: 10.4324/9781003759034-3

encounters, the ideals and hopes of social change, the crazy grandeur that is embedded in every young person and a good dose of naivety kept me together and defined me. Politics gave me a role and a purpose. Meanwhile, common sense and respect for others, acquired phylogenetically, protected me from the violent and extreme tendencies that affected many of my peers at the time. Finally, the Faculty of Medicine shaped me as a person through the discovery of the body, every single muscle and nerve, and the increasingly fascinating and mysterious study of mental functioning.

Encounters are the salt of any story worth telling and that really determine the events of our existence. I remember a teenager, Maria Vittoria, whom I met in the late 1970s while working in Guardia II, the psychiatric ward of Milan's Policlinico University hospital. She was just under 18 years old and was admitted for a dissociative episode, a psychotic onset. She ended up in the room assigned to me, I followed her during her hospitalisation, and we soon began psychoanalytic psychotherapy with three sessions a week. I still remember how engaging it was to work with her. I jealously guard the clinical material and detailed reports of the sessions. After some time, Maria Vittoria decided to change therapists and look for an analyst with more experience than me. She wanted to undergo "real psychoanalysis". I shared and understood her decision, even though I was sorry to see her go. That experience certainly had a profound and positive impact on me, as well as influencing my subsequent professional choices.

In the wake of that encounter – one must find mentors to understand adolescents – I had another one, with Tommaso Senise. He was a Neapolitan "little man", a doctor and anti-fascist who had grown up with historical figures of the city, such as Anna Maria Ortese and Raffaele La Capria, and quoted Eduardo De Filippo in his writings. In the 1950s, after being appointed to the Paolo Pini Psychiatric Hospital, he moved to Milan. Here he met Cesare Musatti, with whom he began psychoanalysis before becoming a psychoanalyst himself. He felt confined within the walls of the psychiatric hospital, where he lived with his family, as was customary at the time. And he began to take care of the most difficult of the boys, those who had committed crimes, almost accidentally it seemed, but for reasons deeply rooted in his own adolescence. He developed an extremely effective methodology of intervention, with insights and innovative aspects that psychoanalysis would accept only after some time, thus becoming one of the pioneers in the treatment of adolescents, a true master, above all of modesty, humility and competence.

The following episode is a perfect illustration of his unmeasurable greatness. I had been admitted to a training group that he led. One day I presented the clinical case of a young woman.

She was a patient who gave me a hard time, but at the same time taught me a lot. She was a curious girl, she asked questions, and she did not passively accept the therapeutic relationship I was proposing to her. I remember that to convince her of the effectiveness of the treatment, I advised her to read *Les mots pour le dire* (1975) [*The Words to Say It*, Italian translation

1984], in which Marie Cardinal recounts her own analysis. Senise had followed my intervention in silence and with great attention. In the end, with his characteristic delicacy, he invited me to interpret what was happening with the patient more carefully. Obviously, in the next session, I followed his instructions to the letter. After a day, the girl ran away from home by train and was found in Rome in a state of confusion. I hadn't related her breakdown to my interpretations. In the next supervision session, however, Tommaso did, by stating: "I was clearly wrong, I gave you the wrong advice, I'm sorry."

And here both a patient and a colleague are united in the genesis of my story as a therapist.

I always say that it is not mandatory to work with adolescents; others can do it just as well. At the same time, it is important to be motivated and passionate.

Young people have very keen perceptions of the authenticity of who is there to help them and relate to them. You can't get anywhere without love and genuine interest when you are dealing with adolescents.

It was quite easy for me to start working with young people. My adolescence still dwelt close in me, having lived it intensely and fully. My emotional world was filled with the moods and flavours of that season of life. I very clearly distinguished between the endless night-time chats with my friends from my youth – some of whom were troubled and problematic – and the first young patients I began to meet in my profession, but the echo and nostalgia of those nights certainly resonated candidly within me.

One question particularly intrigued me. How to find the necessary position between a child's point of view and that of its parents, possibly without upsetting everyone. I decided that I had to listen without prejudice. No one was guilty, everyone was right, it was enough to try to understand the other's point of view and reflect on it together.

Some *out-of-the-box* people I met during my psychoanalytic training were decisive.

I remember I took part in an intensive analytical psychodrama over a weekend with a psychoanalyst of Argentine origin, together with other young colleagues. I still compare it more to an experiential theatre seminar than to an analytical session. One of the sessions dealt with the themes of separation and growth, staged through arguments and discussions that ended with one of the subjects leaving and slamming a door shut. The leader, I almost remember the tone of his words, told us with heartfelt calmness: "Remember that this is an illusory separation. Every door that is slammed shut carries the promise of a door that will have to be reopened. An act of vehemence is not enough to be independent!"

As the years passed, I grew also up. I never stopped feeling close to teenagers, but becoming a father myself made me increasingly accommodating and understanding towards the parents of my young patients. Then, in the natural cycle of life, I began to deal with my own children's adolescence. And that's when I truly understood the struggles my parents had faced in the past. And those of my children in having a parent "competent" in teenagers.

I remember one occasion when I was preparing a report, sitting at the dining room table, with a computer in front of me and lots of books around me. It was evening, and the children, as usual, had taken refuge in their rooms. Suddenly, I felt my daughter's presence behind me.

"What are you doing, Dad?" she asked in a surprisingly interested and curious tone.

"I'm preparing a paper on sexuality in adolescence…", I replied, hoping for openness.

Absolute silence.

After a few moments, I turned around, just in time to see her walking away and saying: "You don't understand anything about teenagers!"

No one is a prophet in their own land.

Despite this harsh judgement, I haven't stopped dealing with adolescents.

Why do I continue?

Firstly, because I enjoy it and get pleasure from it. Secondly, because thanks to them, I feel young and continue to learn. I realised long ago that without my young patients, I wouldn't know almost anything about new music trends, videos, fashions, games, idioms and words that only they know how to invent.

They give me energy and vitality.

I often put myself in their shoes and wonder what goes through their minds when, after more or less reluctantly agreeing to go and talk to a shrink, they find themselves in front of this "old man" in a suit and tie with whom they must spend time and tell their personal stories. I am almost surprised that they come and stay in the room. Every time, I feel a great deal of admiration, a little tenderness and a lot of understanding for their courage and their open willingness to meet me, talk to me and listen to me.

Adolescents enrich the room bringing with them numerous aspects typical of their youth.

Strength and good looks, friendliness and empathy, enthusiasm, the desire to discover, learn and experience. Love, intense feelings, real or imagined tragedies, joys, excitement. A wide variety of objects and tools, backpacks laden with hard work.

Along with many discontinuities, absences, escapes, refusals, oppositions and silences.

Their aromas also enter, sometimes the scent of a season that is about to blossom, amid surprises and anxieties.

The bodies arrive. Lopsided, uncertain, wobbly, cumbersome, like trees that have suddenly grown but do not yet have firm and secure roots. And along with the bodies come the clothes, which often speak much more about them than words.

Or undressed bodies arrive. And I am not referring to the Bermuda shorts, T-shirts and summer sandals of the boys. It is the girls who show me – as they do on the street, in clubs or at school – their skimpy clothes. There is very little consciously seductive about their "undressing", but certainly the body becomes the protagonist of the scene once again. My age and my experience help me to freely voice my emotions, thoughts and even the turmoil that such encounters generate. Thus, it is possible to talk about shapes, disharmony, inadequacies, fears and comparisons – as if it were a Miss Italy beauty contest – but also about beauty, or rather, about harmony which, when it is there, must be mentioned, and when it is lacking, must be sought and found.

Everything that patients bring into the room is a precious gift. What adolescents bring is even more so, like rough diamonds that need to be jealously guarded and valued.

I truly believe that to do this job well, you don't need to feel like you're the "best", but you do need a good dose of intellectual honesty and frankness, as teenagers teach us. Mixed with self-criticism, self-irony and understanding of one's own moods. As befits an adult.

Thanks to encounters with adolescents, psychoanalysis has also changed.

The first and most famous adolescent in psychoanalysis was Dora, an 18-year-old girl seen and described by Freud in 1901. Many therapists specialising in adolescence have since criticised the handling of the case – which was discontinued after only three months of treatment – for the excessive attention given to the point of view and position of the girl's father.

Thirty-five years later, Freud himself met another 18-year-old girl, Margarethe Walter. In 2006, she, the last surviving Freudian patient, recalled in an interview that the then elderly analyst welcomed her into his office at 19 Berggasse in Vienna. He asked some questions, which her father always answered. Freud went silent. Suddenly, he said to Mr Walter in a friendly tone, as if it were the most natural thing in the world: "Please go into the next room. I would like to speak to your daughter alone." He turned his chair towards her, approached her and said openly: "Now we are alone," and immediately the tension eased. And she talked and talked.

"He fulfilled my lifelong desire to open up to someone for the first time: Sigmund Freud was the first person who really showed interest in me, who wanted to know something about me, the only one who really listened to me."

An encounter that changed her life forever.

I believe this is the transformative, even restorative, experience that every teenager would like to have in our offices, the reason why they come and stay with us for as long as necessary.

Annibale – Monday, 4.45 p.m.[1]

My name is Annibale, I am 19 years old.

I don't know why my parents gave me the name of this ancient military leader, Hannibal.

Apparently, they initially wanted to call me Tizio or Caio. I got off lightly.

My younger brother is called Svevo. Psychoanalysis is a family affair. My mother has been in therapy all her life.

Dad isn't, he doesn't talk to anyone, let alone a stranger.

I went back to my shrink because last time, last year, he told me I could do it whenever I wanted, if I had bad things, or even good things, to say. Better yet, to deposit, because it's not that I haven't already said them to someone or processed them in some way, but here, in this room, the words really stay where I put them. And then I find them again. The fact is that since July, a lot of messed up things have happened to me. First the G8 in Genoa, then the new school after two years, the Twin Towers, and I even broke up with my girlfriend. As if that weren't enough, a friend of mine tried to kill herself and after taking the pills she called me. I had to rush over, help her, tell her mum who didn't know who to blame and gave me an endless telling-off. And then, speaking of parents, I realised that in my group of old friends, we all have problems with our fathers. Some have not been recognised, some have been disowned, some are the children of Red Brigade members who are in prison. In the end, perhaps I am the most normal one.

When I first went to a shrink seven years ago, I was almost 13; she was a woman, a friend of my mother's analyst. She interviewed me, gave me tests, and decided that I should continue therapy with a man.

"Because of you, I have to go to another idiot after you," I said when she made this suggestion.

So here I am.

However, it was true that I wasn't well. I had difficulty relating to my peers and didn't know why. Primary school had been great, I was in a protected environment; in short, everything was fine. Then, in secondary school, they enrolled me in a school near my home, in a suburb. Can you imagine the Bronx in New York? Well, it's like that! I would leave school and there would be cars burning – I'll explain later how much they still scare me.

I was pissed off at the time. I was angry with my parents because they didn't take care of me, because they had a lot of work and I hardly ever saw them in the evenings.

I made it clear that I didn't really want to do sessions.

Anyway, I went to see this new psychiatrist, introduced myself, and talked about myself.

I don't even know why, but I couldn't stop talking: about sports, about competitive surfing – my dad always loved that – and then about football, which I played and followed as a fan.

"I'm a fan of Milan. I understand that you are an Inter fan, but that's not a problem."

"I used to play football too. I was a goalkeeper," he said.

I liked that story.

"So, you can put up with everything I say," I replied.

"Maybe you like the idea of being a goalkeeper because he has a net behind him: if things go wrong, it can collect the shots he didn't save."

"Nice idea," I thought, even though I didn't quite understand what he meant.

I liked this first meeting, but I was afraid I had talked too much.

There was a crazy kid at my school who went to a psychologist; everyone said he was crazy precisely because he went to a psychologist, so I didn't tell anyone and I stopped talking, even during interviews.

After six sessions, I stopped going.

Two years later, at the age of 15, I went back on my own initiative, partly to see what it was like, partly out of curiosity. Maybe I needed it, but I don't think I had more than a few sessions.

By then, I only hung out with people from my neighbourhood on the outskirts of town, and I was always out and about. That's where I got to know and did everything: drugs, dealing, fighting, death. They killed someone like me because he didn't want to deliver stuff for them anymore. I was proud of what was happening to me. I still have a scar on my back. I was proud of it and cherished it. Now I wish I didn't have it anymore.

At that time, we moved out of the city to a large, renovated farmhouse with a courtyard, a sort of twenty-first-century commune, that felt out of time, out of place. And high school was a real disaster: I started dealing every drug I could get my hands on. I needed money because I was doing a gram of amphetamine a day to keep up with the joints and smoking. I had a lot of disposable girlfriends; I destroyed everyone around me. And, as expected, I left school.

I don't think I'd still be here if I hadn't met Pino, an adult friend, at some point. He was my salvation. He taught me how to draw, how to enjoy peace and quiet, how to make myself tea and biscuits at four in the afternoon and how to go to bed early. He was the adult I needed, without being my father.

So, I went back to the shrink a couple of times after another two years – I was 17 by then – but I didn't really say anything. Again.

By then I had enrolled in art school, I was going to community centres, I was involved in politics. Everything seemed fine, except that I failed my exams, perhaps because of a sort of pit stop – a pause button – in my life, and I decided to tell my parents everything that had happened since middle school. I told my mum to hurt her, and my dad to make him feel excluded, just as he had always excluded me. I felt terrible. For a fortnight, I didn't understand anything anymore. So, I looked for my shrink, and the bastard was on holiday from the end of July to September. That summer, I had met Fausta, a psychologist ten years older than me, and I had started a relationship with her, even though she already had someone else. In short, I was really messed up.

Finally, in September, I saw the psychiatrist again. And I told him everything: about the drugs and everything else. That things were getting worse and worse at home, everyone was against me, no one in the courtyard could stand me anymore, I was taking space away from my brother. I felt like shit.

Two days later, I called the doctor in tears.

"I want to leave home for a few days." He agreed, proposing a deal.

"All right, just don't take any drugs."

He couldn't have known that I was already past that phase, but his words were very important to me. I felt that they were close to my heart and necessary, just as I felt that he understood me, cared about me and set limits for me. Could we say that he loved me?

I was away from home for a fortnight, then I came back; I was still feeling bad, but this time my mother helped me, she took me around to find a private school where I could do two years paying tuition, and it really helped me. The sessions lasted a few months, then when I felt better, I stopped. That year I passed my exams.

Then there was Genoa, the G8.

It seemed like a great opportunity, something peaceful and fun, with friends.

Even now, when I talk about it, I feel like dying, they attacked us immediately, splitting the procession in two, coming at us from all sides while helicopters circled overhead. I seriously thought I wouldn't make it. And perhaps it was precisely because of that fear that I started attacking, charging, throwing stones, bottles, anything I could get my hands on. I took a lot and gave a lot. I was pure adrenaline, I didn't recognise myself anymore and neither did my friends. There are photos of me in the newspapers, I appear in television footage, because I was there too, charging and burning the police van, and I was there just before they killed Carlo Giuliani. I could have been in his place if I hadn't run away in time.

I was left with the taste of a great political defeat, a sense of discouragement, of failure. I was already on the train back to Milan when I heard that they had attacked the Diaz school, although I hadn't yet heard of how brutal that raid was. The next day I was back in the square crying from the tear gas, but none of us did anything sensational.

I think I was traumatised, I talked about it all the time: some people treated me like a hero, and it drove me crazy. A hero? I was scared shitless; I don't even know what I had done!

I enjoyed talking about it, telling him everything, it felt like I could finally leave this story in a safe place. Even now, I wake up at night with nightmares, I see terrible images in front of me, I relive that day on the front line with terror. I could talk about it for days and days.

I also changed schools; I had to get used to it. Fausta and I broke up after she finally left the other guy. But it's for the best, it's better, we have different needs. But we're still friends.

And then my friend attempted suicide.

And the Twin Towers. I thought it was a film!

"That's why I came back here, and now I'd like to stay for a while. May I?"

What stopped me from destroying the shrink?

The first time because I was afraid of that horrible wizard.

The second time because I was afraid that he would tell me I was mad.

Then because I discovered and loved psychology and the books he recommended to me.

Finally, because he has a beautiful office and a lovely, friendly wife with a laughing voice.

"Isn't your wife the colleague you share your office with?"

After the dream I left on the answering machine the other night, I felt too exposed again, too forward.

"What are we doing here? I'm not going on that couch, I'm not ready. I know I'll have therapy sooner or later, especially if I do your job. But I'd like to work with children, because I like drawing and playing and so…"

Of course, things have changed! I no longer need to feel like God to feel good; I'm letting go of my beliefs and it's a good thing because they were ungrounded. I believe that to understand your limits, you must try everything, to measure yourself against them in a head-to-head battle.

I think you leave childhood behind when you realise that your parents have flaws.

And that you leave adolescence behind when you accept these flaws.

Returning to the room was a bit like seeing a friend again, a loved one, someone you had left behind but who had always been there. Like those friendships where seeing each other again after a long time is like picking up a conversation left unfinished the day before.

Well, it's the same with my therapist.

So, I told him about myself, my plans, my difficulties, my fears and my successes. It seemed to me that he felt as if they were his, but he never stole them from me, he took them in and then gave them back to me.

It wasn't easy to be close to me, to accompany me through all these years.

It has been difficult for many people.

I'm sorry if I hurt anyone. This has been my life. For now.

I've been told that psychologists are very happy when they can find out what happens over the years to the people they have treated. It even has a name, it's called catamnesis. It helps them to better understand how to treat people. To do research. To improve.

For my part, I've changed my mind so often that sometimes I've lost myself too.

Even now I still don't really know who I am or what I want.

I only know that at a certain point I had to grow up, and I realised that I would have to add a chapter to the sequences of life which I don't think will be the last.

I think you become an adult when you must deal with your parents' flaws.

When I became an adult, I decided it was also time to pay for the sessions myself. The shrink was kind enough to give me a nice discount and last time he even wrote my story and gave it to me. It's this.

I was pleased; I found it interesting. I haven't seen him since then.

But I must confess that I didn't pay him for the last two sessions. Could this be a way to go back, sooner or later?

Greta – Tuesday, 1.45 p.m.

It all started one night. That night.

When I was little, it was always my critical moment. As soon as it got dark, when they turned off the light, the hard part began for me. Fear? We can call it that. Like a slow but inexorable flow rising to my throat, blocking my thoughts, paralysing my words. Loneliness. I felt totally alone, abandoned, lost. Where had my mum gone? Who was my dad? Who would ever come looking for me? I didn't know, and falling asleep terrified me.

A rag doll and a night light made it bearable until I was eight. Then I found a sense of security and trust. I slept well.

Until that summer night, the last of my thirteenth year.

The day after was my milestone birthday.

I was calm, sleeping soundly, school behind me, the weekend approaching and the holidays not far off. Suddenly, a sharp pain in my side woke me with a start. I tried to turn over in bed, changed position, waited a little. Nothing. The pain doesn't go away, it gets more intense, it expands to my whole stomach. I start to get scared. I don't want to call my parents; I don't want to disturb them. They already have their own struggles. In addition to those of previous years, when it really seemed to me that they had lost their way a little. My mother tried to get the family back together and, in the meantime, became a doormat, then an ornament, now a person again. My dad is tired; he travels a lot for work. I'm sorry. I try to distract myself with these memories, with thoughts, but nothing works, the pain is still there.

OK, I'll call my mum.

She knows me, she knows I don't make a fuss about nothing, that I'm quite brave. A lively and cheerful child, a model student with a sunny personality. That's my portrait. Lots of interests, lots of friends. I like psychology and martial arts. Even though I'm small, I'm tough.

She looks at me, understands, wakes up my dad, the emergency room is just a few minutes away. Code yellow. Waiting.

The diagnosis is peritonitis, not exactly reassuring. But they don't operate on me urgently. I am admitted to an adult ward without my mum. Like Gandhi, she engages in passive resistance and sleeps on the floor next to my bed. She's tough too, no doubt about it.

Here another story begins, with all kinds of implications: medical, surgical, even legal.

Can I summarise it without too many details? The memory still hurts. They call it trauma.

I have the operation on Monday morning, complications arise, the operation lasts longer than expected, they keep me in hospital for six days, I leave and my fever rises, an infection, new surgery, drainage for three weeks, daily dressings, pain.

My parents argue with the doctors.

I get my first period on the day of the operation. Call it coincidence?

When I return home, I continue to feel pain and have difficulty walking. My right leg gives way.

"My leg has come back!" I say for a long time to make myself understood.

I feel ill, I am agitated. Sometimes the agitation becomes intense, especially when I think about being hospitalised. I have nightmares.

What is happening to me? What have they done to me?

So, America becomes a pipe dream and a solution: that's where the solution is, they will finally understand everything and cure me for sure. Instead, the diagnosis arrives: I have suffered a nerve compression injury, but this does not explain the pain and motor impairment. The subtext is that I also need psychological help.

And here I am.

At first, I am wary and I bare my claws. I am very aggressive. I know it and I do nothing to hide it. I did not want to come to therapy. I do not want to be in need. But I could not oppose my mother either. And then I do not like men, they scare me, especially doctors. They all seem violent, intrusive and destructive to me. Like the boys I have relationships with, who run away, or those who chase after me, exhibitionists and disrespectful. Not to mention my father, who hasn't looked at me since I got sick.

I want to be independent; I don't want to depend on anyone. Is that clear?

The truth is that I don't recognise myself. I used to be sweet, kind, I knew how to be with people. But I have been completely overthrown by everything that has happened since the operation, totally changing the situation, turning my functioning mechanisms upside down, inverting the relationship between reason and feelings. Feelings are not exactly my strong point; they never have been.

So, little by little, I try to be good, now that I'm here, I try to fit in.

The doctor wants to know everything about my past, the operation, how I felt, what I experienced. The facts, but also my feelings. This is new for me.

I talk easily, but above all I listen to words I've never heard before.

"Dear Greta, you are a curious person, but you have an immense control over your emotions and feelings. It seems that your emotions are mysteries to you, especially when it comes to anger and rage. You are also a kind person; I can understand it from the words you use to describe things."

Upon hearing these words, I slowly begin to thaw. He explains to me that I try to keep unpleasant emotions at bay by resorting to rationality, associated with control. Some people are more inclined to reflection and getting in contact with their emotions. Yet I find it easier to keep everything inside and at a distance, but he imagines that I know that the situation is much more complex than it appears at first glance.

In short, I am going through a very delicate moment in my life, and perhaps I would not be there, in that room, if a series of events had not happened all at once. First, I have no familiarity with emotions. Then all the medical issues with all that they entailed. Finally, something more delicate, concerning my father: I was very close to my dad, and this bond, he explains, as often happens with daughters, changed when I grew up and stopped being the little girl I once was. It happens that fathers, especially when faced with the physical changes in their daughters, struggle to find a new way of being together. Not to mention the onset of menstruation, with all its real and symbolic consequences. His hypothesis is that these emotional and physical changes have overwhelmed me.

"You might ask me now: what does all this have to do with your leg that sometimes doesn't work? Excellent question! I confess that I don't know but trying to answer it could be a good reason to meet up, talk about what's happening to you, understand you better, get to know you a little more. What do you say? What do you think about what I've told you?"

My first reaction to his speech is rather impulsive: a bit long-winded, don't you think?

My second reaction is more articulate: don't psychoanalysts always keep quiet? Once you give this guy the floor, no one can take it away from him.

Third. More thoughtful. I liked what he said, but I don't say so explicitly, perhaps because I'm not even sure myself. I agree to see him again, to give us and him some time. I'm convinced. I'll give it a try, at least.

I get up from my chair to head for the exit.

After a couple of steps, suddenly, my leg gives way, as it often does, as I have known for some time, but this time it gets me off guard, I am about to fall to the ground.

The doctor catches me. First with one hand, as if to offer me support. Then with the other, to accompany me. There is no music, no orchestra or band, not even a CD playing in the background, but I feel like I'm starting to dance. Together. A waltz, swirling skirts, hair blowing in the wind, a tulle tutu, a double step, happy and light. On the other hand, ten years of ballet, albeit abruptly interrupted by my "leg", are not easily forgotten. When we reach the door, I have already regained my balance on one leg, like a crane, and I hop over to my mother in the waiting room. At ease, serene, without shame.

The dances, evidently, have begun.

They will continue for a long time, with a few difficulties, but with great satisfaction.

In time, I will become a good dancer. And I will dance alone.

Antonio – No Day, No Time

Locked in my room, sitting on the floor, legs crossed, chest upright, hands cupped one on top of the other, a small smile on my lips, eyes closed. I seek comfort.

I begin.

I like to feel my body resting on the ground, the feeling of having something solid beneath me gives me security.

I try to release tension, both muscular and mental. If I remember, I smile too, it relaxes me.

I am ready. I breathe.

Breathing is normal; we wouldn't be able to live without it. It's the first thing we do when we're born.

The amount of air that is inhaled during the very first breath is more important than during any subsequent breath in your life. Here I am already getting distracted.

I breathe.

Air enters me. Air leaves me.

I feel it in my nostrils. I feel it on my lips. I feel it in my chest. I feel it in my belly.

I breathe.

I don't strain, I don't force, I let it happen. It happens.

I don't think. I try.

Thoughts.

They don't go away, they continue to arise incessantly, invading me, distracting me.

I notice them. Awareness. I smile. At myself, at my mind, at my commitment.

I brush them away, like waving my hand at an annoying fly.

I breathe.

How much time has passed? More thoughts, more distractions. More attention.

I breathe.

Like this, without respite, without anguish, without pain, without effort.

Like a mountain stream that continues to flow incessantly. Without noise, without anything. Without.

Fifteen minutes are enough for me. I'm done, I'm almost sorry, I feel good. I'm happy.

Tomorrow again.

In recent months, I have become accustomed to practising this way, which is how mindfulness entered my life. Every day for a few minutes – ten to 15 – there is no need to be fanatical and spend hours on it. It is a small companion, a habit. At first, I followed an audio track, but now I can do it on my own. I've got used to it, perhaps I've learned it. I can feel it. I do it. Just like that.

How did it all start? Let's take a small step back.

At my age, already 16 years old, I would really prefer to have a better life. Without psychologists, I hope.

I've been there before, I even liked it a little, then it went wrong. Enough.

My life, big words, bro! I don't want to go to any shrinks, but I'm not doing so well now and I'd like some help, I don't know from whom.

My parents are helping me. They're at my service, I'd say. I'm always grateful to them.

Driving, outside contacts, phone calls, school changes, various plans.

Without them, I wouldn't be able to do anything. They are made of iron; they never give up.

They decided to go to a psychoanalyst who works with young people and doesn't expect me to go with them. He saw them, spoke to their GP, and they decided on a course of treatment. Medication, for now.

I'm taking pills. Let's hope they don't hurt me.

In fact, I hope they do me good.

I'm almost always shut up at home. I'm not a *hikikomori*, one of those Japanese people who live with their computer in their room and a tray of food outside their door. But I do spend a lot of time on the computer. The game is called *League of Legends* and it's very popular in Italy, but even more so around the world (in Korea it's considered a sport in all respects). It's very competitive, so it takes a lot of practice to improve. Anyway, one of the few moments when I feel free is when I'm in front of the screen: I stop thinking and focus only on the game.

Oh well, since I'm here, I'll try writing to him. If he's different, he'll reply.

> *Good morning, this is Antonio. I know you spoke to my parents. I am writing to you because I am not feeling well now and I would like your help. I often have this feeling of not being in myself, as if I were looking at my body from the outside. I keep thinking about it. Sometimes I've felt ill, I didn't understand what was going on around me and I had a panic attack. So, I often have trouble going out because I'm afraid it might happen again, since I think about this feeling all the time. For over a week now, I've only been going out with my mum and in the car because I feel like it's a safe place. All this is making my life very difficult. I often don't go to school. I'm afraid it might happen to me there too. I also felt ill one evening in the countryside. I was outside with the dog, looking at the stars and thinking about infinity, how far away the stars were, and suddenly I felt ill. It was as if I were falling into a ravine. These thoughts of infinity, of the sky and the world in general, affect me deeply. I started having these fears, these fears of feeling ill, about two years ago. At times I go out, although I always have limitations, while at other times I am stuck at home. One thing I can no longer stand is crowded or particularly large places. When I enter a closed environment, I always look for the exit, it makes me feel calmer. A small remedy I have found for when I am a little more agitated is to pinch my legs. It helps me focus on the pain rather than my feelings. Sometimes I have taken photos of myself while I looked to the right or left to confirm that my eye was moving, and I often touch my head to make sure I still have it. I feel quite ridiculous. The fact is, it seems strange to me how two little eyes can have such a wide field of vision. Thinking about these things bothers me. Even writing this email makes me a little nervous. I hope I have been clear enough about my situation and I hope you can help me!:-).*

Rereading this, I realise I've gone a bit overboard. What am I looking for? Hope, I suppose.

In the meantime, a reply will suffice. Clear, respectful. And maybe it won't even arrive. How do I know if this guy is into long-distance relationships? Will he answer me, or won't he? Who cares…

Instead, two days go by, and here's his email.

> *Dear Antonio, what you are experiencing has a very clear name: panic attacks. A panic attack is an acute disorder that starts with very intense anxiety and subsequently becomes a thought disorder. During a panic attack, our thoughts lead us to believe that terrible things could happen to us, even death. Often, those who have suffered from panic attacks subsequently develop a phenomenon that seems very similar to what you are experiencing: anticipatory fear of having a panic attack. At times, this fear can cause even greater suffering than the attack itself. It is essential that you first understand and develop this concept: the fear of having a panic attack is just a thought. There is a profound difference between having a panic attack and thinking you are going to have a panic attack. First, I would like you to reflect on this concept and internalise the difference between thought and event. The second thing is to establish a treatment…*

Here I begin to be less convinced. I have already said that I do not want to see any "shrink-something". I take medication and that's fine. Going to therapy, even a different kind, does not convince me. I do not want to think or understand.

I just want to feel good! Now. Immediately. And I don't want to see anyone. Is that clear?

But he was kind. I reply. Calmly, but I reply.

> *Hello, you reassured me about my thoughts, I thought I was going mad! Regarding therapy, however, I'm a little scared. Just thinking about how I feel creates a lot of problems for me, so I don't think I can go to someone and describe them, because it would almost certainly make me feel ill and it would cause me just as much anxiety. For the same reason, I can't come to see you in person. Feeling ill in my own room makes me worry much less than feeling ill in other places. Is there anything I can do at home to try to reduce these feelings and fears? Who knows, maybe by taking small steps at a time…*

Answer.

> *Yes, there is one thing. It involves guided meditation practices, the purpose of which is… not to think… Ideally, you would take a beginner's course, but you don't want to do anything, do you? However, you could look at this website:* tempomindfulness.com. *Or read and use these two books:* The Art and Science of Mindfulness *(with a CD) and* Mindfulness for Beginners. *Then we'll talk about it…*

Mindfulness? What's that? It sounds like something for old people or weirdos. For people who have time to waste or don't know how to spend their time. Maybe it could be useful for my mother. She's stressed, always rushing around. Between cleaning and things to do, work and family. Poor thing, I understand her.

But what have I got to lose? I've got plenty of time. It's not like I have a list of commitments and outings to tick off. Come on, I'll give it a try. If it doesn't work, I'll stop!

Thus, a new phase began.

> *I read the book and identified with many parts of it. But I don't understand how a little breathing can get me out of this situation, taking away all these thoughts/paranoia/fears. But if you assure me that you can help me overcome all this thanks to the CD, I will do it. It's been a month since I started taking alprazolam and I also want to know what to do now. In fact, something has changed because now I am beginning to feel more or less calm, better every day. So, if these breathing exercises can help me, I will do them gladly. If the medicine helps me take a few small steps to gradually get out of this, I would be happy.*

Because I'm stubborn. If I set my mind on something and I like it, I do it. I kept going, partly because Doc encouraged me.

> *It's true, you must believe in what I'm proposing. But if you really practise every day, after a month or so you'll start to see the first benefits.*

After a month, I wrote to him again.

> *I am happily continuing my mindfulness practice. I have noticed that the breathing exercises help me keep my mind distracted when I need it most. The exercises on sounds and thoughts bother me a little more. I followed the exercises on some websites and the ones in the book. I always tried to do the ones that lasted no more than 25 minutes, because otherwise they start to weigh on me and I do them reluctantly, whereas I happily do the 15–20–25-minute ones in a day. I find some exercises difficult to understand; this awareness is not yet clear to me. Probably what I need most is to practise accepting thoughts and welcoming them, not harping on them, but just looking at them as mental events. I think this is the key to my problem. However, I cannot fully grasp this concept of awareness. I know they are just thoughts, but they frighten me and cause me bad feelings anyway. One thing I have noticed about myself is that if I feel like going for a ride on my motorbike or a walk during the day, my mind almost unconsciously tells me: remember that you suffer from panic attacks, and then I start to get a little scared. It is as if I want to go out, but the fear of feeling ill prevents me from doing so. Another thing I've noticed is that I*

find it easier to do things as soon as I leave school or after doing some activity, whereas if I tell myself I'll go out for a walk in an hour, I find it more difficult. Doing things without thinking about them is much easier for me than doing things I've planned.

The doctor was thrilled.

Hello Antonio. I was very pleased to receive your email. I am very flattered by what you wrote and by the progress you are making. I admire your intelligence and your ability to use the stimuli you are given. I am very happy with what you are doing and how you are doing. What is happening to you is exactly what I hoped would happen and what I hoped you would be able to do. You just need to continue the path you have started. Achieving these results and this awareness in such a short time is a very positive indication of the effectiveness of the work. Don't worry if you struggle to exceed 25 minutes, that's more than enough.

I am also very happy. Even though I am struggling terribly, I am never satisfied.

I replied.

Now I'm afraid that the improvements will disappear, that I'll feel bad again, that everything will vanish.

He replied too. He doesn't always do it straight away; he takes his time. I understand.

They say you should always leave sometime between writing an email and sending it; they've even written some little rules about it. I don't follow any of them; it's back and forth. Action, reaction. Or I never reply. I'm not a millennial for nothing!

It is precisely this aspect that I would like to focus on. The effort. I understand how painful it is for you to feel that the things you have achieved may vanish. It is painful and disappointing. On the other hand, each of us achieves progress and evolution by trying and trying again. If we do not dare, we will never change, we will never improve! Obviously, this also becomes a bit risky, according to the old proverb that says, "Those who leave the old road for the new know what they are leaving, but not what they will find." We could call it courage, curiosity, experimentation. It should come natural at your age, if you manage it serenely. What I would like to offer you is a slightly different perspective on your fears. I don't know if you have any experience or knowledge of mountains and climbing. People who climb mountains do so in stages and in different steps. In big climbs, these are called base camp and advanced camps. Very often, you reach a higher camp and then you may have to descend for various reasons. It may seem like giving up or a waste of time. In reality, on the one hand, it is necessary to acclimatise, and on the other, climbing back up to a camp you have already reached is less difficult because the route has already been traced, but above all because we know we have already travelled it and therefore are confident that it is possible and that we can do it. A good and secure foundation! But let's imagine the worst-case scenario. You climb the mountain for a while and then you slip and find yourself lower down. Of course, afterwards you may feel frightened, disappointed and tired. However, once you have recovered, you should find a sense of security inside yourself: you had already been able to reach the point from which you slipped during the ascent!

Interesting.

I didn't tell him that I immediately thought that when you fall you could also hurt yourself. For once, I thought positively, I didn't want to be a "downer".

Anyway, a new thought immediately sprang to mind. Every now and then, I feel like a factory of thoughts.

Should I write? Yes, I will.

Hello, I am pleased with the message I received, but now I have another worry on my mind. I have already told you that I spend a lot of time playing on the computer. Now I am concerned that I may be addicted to gaming and that it is distracting me from the important things in life. I play more or less every day, for a total of five or six hours. It's what I think about most during the day, which means that I spend most of my time thinking about this game, afraid that it might become addictive or obsessive and that this virtual world might take the place of my real world and make it difficult for me to interact with other people, and not give priority to the most important things. I don't know if this is just my paranoia or something real that could cause me problems. Probably I'm not explaining myself so that you can understand but I hope I managed to convey it to you, because I tried my best. Thank you very much and I hope to hear from you soon!

Response.

Dear Antonio, thank you for your sincerity and transparency. These are uncommon qualities. You have already described the problem perfectly. Using a computer for many hours a day, whatever you do, is addictive and risks blocking thoughts and energy in an obsessive way. Meditation should also serve to break these vicious circles. There are two ways to do this. You can set time limits (defining a maximum amount of time per day for using the computer), even if it means losing your ranking. Or you can quit altogether, like someone addicted to alcohol, smoking or drugs. Let's start by seeing how you react to these suggestions.

I imagined as much. I have a problem. Gosh, I hadn't realised until now. I've made up my mind. Now I'm going to commit myself and give it my all. At least I'll try. After a while, I wanted to tell him.

> *This week, I've cut down to about three hours a day. Is that enough, or should I cut down even more?*

It's not like he congratulated me, I know I'm only just starting.

> *Well, at least three hours of gaming, plus the rest… it's not really that little. But, I'd say, let's be satisfied with that for now.*

However, little by little, the situation began to change.

I could hardly contain my joy. I shared it.

> *Things are going well for now. I'm doing things that I couldn't even imagine a few months ago (going out for a bit with my friends and going on quite long motorbike rides with my mum following behind in the car), and all this is definitely giving me a better outlook on life, as I slowly start doing the things I enjoy and have always done. I have also reduced the amount of time I spend on the computer and now I know that my fear of becoming obsessed with video games is not true because, after an hour and a half in the afternoon, I got tired of playing and I wanted to go out. When I go out and do things I enjoy, my mind hardly ever wanders to the game and, in the evening, yes, I want to play, but it is also true that I have a lot of time to fill. Obviously, it's a game I like and enjoy, but it's not the only thing that I enjoy. If I had the opportunity to go out with my friends or go for a ride on my motorbike, I would immediately leave the game and go and do that.*

I was pretty sure about the applause. By now, I understand what he likes.

> *As always, your thoughts are very clear and understandable. The irritation that your thoughts produce in you, as you describe in a previous email you sent me, depends on the fact that sometimes, as in this case, they take on a circular and repetitive pattern. This makes you feel trapped in circles of thought, like running around in circles around a pole, and you don't know how to get out of it. Overall, however, it demonstrates you're able to maintain a commitment with consistency and continuity. You are currently applying this to the computer, but in the future it could be very valuable in different activities and tasks.*

And with spring, the world has changed completely. I wrote to him again.

> *In recent weeks, everything has been going much better for me. I've been out with friends, riding my motorbike (even taking friends places) and I*

> *even went to one of their houses. The sunshine we've had in recent weeks has done me good and brought me satisfaction and happiness.*

In the meantime, I continue to "breathe". Not every day, but when I find the time, when I feel the need, when I get a little lost in my thoughts. Just a few minutes, but good minutes.

As for the doctor, I haven't written to him for a while, but for now I'm satisfied. I don't want to take advantage of him. Each time I wrote to him I was a little afraid he wouldn't reply.

It was strange to ask for help from someone I didn't even know. But I felt close to him, and that he knew me and I knew him. That this was enough, even without ever seeing him. For now. Right?

Anyway, I think one of these days I'll go and see him.

Afraid? Yes, of finding him different from how I imagined him. It's a risk I'll have to take.

There's at least one thing I could do if I saw him, though. Ask him that question I never managed to formulate in my emails, because it was too intimate and direct.

"Out of curiosity, Doctor, what do you know about *mindfulness*? Why did you recommend it to me?"

And I breathe.

The Analyst and Matteo – Tuesday, 3.45 p.m.

He was 16 years old. He was a small but compact, stocky boy, the kind you'd rather not get into a fight with. Those of us who usually deal with the mind often forget about the body. His parents had sent him to therapy. He wasn't very happy about it, but he came to the sessions anyway.

Vague, inconsistent, a liar, a terrible student, a dangerous friend and an unreliable boyfriend, he abused alcohol and drugs. The son of a wealthy family, he lived practically alone, enjoying a level of independence that was completely disproportionate with his age. Having free access to his part of the house, he had turned it into a laboratory for refining, dealing and consuming cocaine and hashish. There was no trace of self-criticism in Matteo; every action was justified, logical and authorised by a grandiose and megalomaniacal self. On the other hand, his parents were unaware of everything, as is often the case. A form of self-protection. Out of sight, out of mind.

I disliked Matteo.

Donald Winnicott, the eminent English paediatrician and psychoanalyst, defined what was happening to me with Matteo in the middle of the last century as "countertransference hatred". Because I really struggled to keep my normative and parental instincts in check. Perhaps even a little sadistically. Matteo certainly seemed like a petulant child, incapable of staying in his place – objectively, no one had ever told him to – which triggered desires for punishment and rules. Emotionally, he seemed to be in disarray. I was no better.

That Tuesday session was no worse than any other. He talked. I listened patiently, perhaps distractedly.

I found it very difficult to be there.

At one point, playing on my emotions after his uncontrollable account of his latest exploits, I pointed out his desire to challenge me, and this exchange began:

"Matteo, look, if we continue this virtual tug-of-war, you're sure to win. But in the end, will there really be a winner?" I was hoping to find some reasonable support.

"If that's the case, I'd win in a real tug-of-war too!"

Until that moment, I had been fully aware of what was happening, but suddenly, like Giuditta inside Roberto Benigni's body in *Il Piccolo Diavolo* [*The Little Devil*] – we can call it the unconscious for simplicity's sake – without realising it, these words came out of my mouth: "I wouldn't take that for granted…"

"Let's see," Matteo replied mockingly.

At that point, I left. Only Giuditta remained on stage.

"Do you want to try? I'm fine with it!"

"OK!" he replied.

I believe that Matteo's physical characteristics, still typically boyish, notwithstanding his being muscular, prompted me to accept the challenge. I was confident of how it would turn out. It was clear that I had to win to be credible. Although it meant overcoming that parental instinct that leads us to play and compete with our children on the hazy confines between commitment and renunciation. We would like them to beat us, but it is only our victory that becomes a healthy reality check for them, an opportunity for growth.

So, we cleared the table and took our positions for what was more of an arm wrestle than a tug-of-war. One arm here, one arm there, elbows aligned, some effort due to the different levers, we clasped hands and began the epic challenge. Those hands, which until then had only clasped in greetings at the end of the session, were now clasped for another reason. The struggle for power, no doubt about it.

I won, perhaps with Giuditta's help.

Now another session and another therapy began here.

I came back to myself. Giuditta had finally left my body.

Matteo was devastated, mortified.

It was the first time that sadness appeared on his face and in his thoughts. He had had to come to terms with his own limitations, thanks to someone who had pointed them out to him, but now was not taking advantage of them.

Now I found it easier to connect with him and, at the same time, rediscover my more welcoming and empathetic sides.

We talked about the battle we had staged. I tried to explain to him what had happened between us, why we had ended up challenging each other "for real" and not just in verbal clashes. What was the meaning and significance of it all? We tried to put it together. I was a little aware, knowing that I also had to come to terms with my unconscious, with those unresolved, if not unknown, areas. Why, I asked myself, was I doing this now if I had never fought with anyone, not even when I was a boy. Matteo accepted this new way of working. But I had set myself on a path fraught with obstacles, with trials that were too complex and risky.

After a certain period in which he had apparently turned into a "good patient", he arrived at the session looking gloomy. It didn't take me long to fall for his provocation. I don't even remember what I said, or didn't say, in response to something he said. Certainly, something that didn't suit him.

And then his anger exploded.

In our profession, we sometimes face aggression, real risks to our physical safety. In the old psychiatric wards and asylums, it was good practice for the doctor to sit near the door, ready to leave if necessary, with the patient on the other side of the room.

That wasn't the case, not in my room. Bad choice in this instance. That day, the storm only hit objects: books, papers, pens, the bin, chairs, my beloved dracaena, everything was targeted by Matteo's destructive fury.

I have never been caught in a tornado or a hurricane; I have only seen footage of them.

In only a few minutes the room looked like a scene from *The Day After Tomorrow*. I couldn't believe it. I was stunned and frightened. I was worried about what would happen next. How would it end?

Matteo quickly regained full control of himself. He sat back down in his chair, he gazed with satisfaction at the spectacle he had created and exhaled a long, deep, almost noisy breath, and looked me straight in the eye. Immediately after flashing me a satisfied smile, he got up and left.

To my relief and sense of liberation.

I did nothing to stop him. I didn't say a word. This hadn't been an uncontrollable and unexpected explosive crisis, typical of psychotic episodes. Matteo's behaviour seemed to be the result of a premeditated plan waiting to be carried out. It seemed as if he had waited for the right moment, the right opportunity. A cold-blooded revenge.

He had only spared me the direct physical consequences. And it certainly wasn't me who stopped him; I think it was more his own choice.

Once the fear of the moment had passed, I had time to think about the events.

I had put our relationship on the level of physical challenge, shifting the confrontation from ideas to that of strength. Maybe I had also taken advantage of the situation because I needed to seize an excuse to "punish" him, perhaps to redirect some of the aggression that was circulating between us. The proverb says, "Those who live by the sword die by the sword." The arm-wrestling challenge was not a good choice, nor was it the only one possible.

I haven't seen Matteo since our last match. An external, neutral referee could determine the winner and loser.

Perhaps he would declare a draw.

I don't care, nor does it console me: we both lost.

Note

1 Taken, with subsequent amendments, from the report presented at the 12th Congress of the Italian Psychoanalytical Society, Trieste, 2002, published in G. Berti Ceroni (ed.), Come cura la psicoanalisi [How Psychoanalysis Heals], Franco Angeli, Milan, 2005.

4 Ginger Candies, Watches and Handkerchiefs

"You don't care about me at all. You're only doing this for the money, for the bank transfer at the end-of-month. Even if I died tomorrow, you wouldn't give a damn."

With these words, Mara broke the silence that had fallen between us towards the end of the session, a seemingly quiet session. I was already in the mood to say goodbye; we just had to agree on some temporary changes to our appointments. Instead...

A gunshot. Words, like bullets, fly in my direction. I dodge them, they don't touch me, but they hurt me deeply. They are imprinted on the wall behind me. I suddenly feel a burning sensation starting on my face, then rushing throughout my body. My heart is beating fast, my hands are shaking, an itch quickly rises my legs to my thighs. I know what transference is, I can guess whose place I am taking. It is a whiplash, a snap close to my face, it hurts. I react indignantly.

"Mara, with all due respect for your thoughts, you cannot know what is going through my mind."

A bad response. Sincere, but bad.

Calmness, time and awareness would have suggested other solutions. A better rapport.

Something like: "Mara, I'm very sorry you feel that way. I don't agree with what you said, but we must accept your thoughts. How about we try to understand together why you have this idea, how it came about and how we can deal with it?" Perhaps it would have allowed us to understand that, among other things, Mara was asking me how important she really was for me.

This is the other side of relationality. Getting deeply and actively involved in therapeutic dynamics can delude us into thinking that being "good and empathetic" is enough to heal others. We forget that discomfort has much deeper and more complex roots, that traumatic ruptures and lack of recognition need time to heal. It takes testing and counter-tests of reciprocal trust, and further and continuous verification. When you have already been burned you live in a state of alertness. And yet, we sometimes risk not tolerating the legitimate and physiologically aggressive and hostile reactions of patients,

DOI: 10.4324/9781003759034-4

which we may experience as betrayal or ingratitude. Instead, we know how necessary and useful it is to feel that you have done what was for the best and that it is a fundamental step in growing and healing. Even when it involves breaking a reassuring balance. Sometimes too reassuring.

Healing, at times, also means "touching" on some sore points. An analysis is a sequence of seemingly repetitive and insignificant episodes. Hence it becomes impossible to expect compelling or riveting scenes as depicted at the cinema.

An average viewer would be bored.

There are times, however, in those special passages that Daniel Stern called "present moments", when something happens that leaves an indelible and definitive mark of transformation. These are events that mark a turning point. It happens when language is not limited to verbally communicating thoughts, but also the feelings and sensations that accompany them.

"After the last session, when I left the building, I felt strange. I sat down on a bench and started to reflect. I don't know why, but I don't feel the same as I did before anymore. I'm fine, but I don't understand. Can you tell me what happened, can you explain what's going on?" Silvia asked me this in the session following one where she had been very upset.

What seems to happen is that you are left with a sort of suspended feeling. It doesn't only happen to the patients, but it happens to me too. Certain sessions have a different feel to them, opening surprising and unexpected scenarios.

When I am fully aware of what has happened, I share it immediately with the patient. Other times, we talk about it later.

It is as if a shift has taken place.

We are here and we find ourselves there, in another space and world, surprised and incredulous, even a little frightened.

The creativity of therapy often lies precisely in the possibility of discovering a new and surprising plan. Many pathologies arise from unconscious repetitions, compulsions, and patterns of behaviour and thought. This profession is so beautiful because it really offers the possibility of having new experiences. Doing it together, building bridges between the past and the present, is exciting and leaves us with a sense of fulfilment. It is like constructing or reassembling a new structure from the fragmented parts of ourselves.

"It was a good session, very intense. A beautiful moment!" recalls Guido.

Something evocative had also happened to him many years previously. We often talked about cinema in our sessions. That day, he was telling me about the emotions he felt when watching *Dead Man Walking* (Tim Robbins, 1995), the story of the encounter between a man sentenced to death and a nun who assists him in the last days of his life. The title is taken from the expression commonly used by American prison guards to announce the journey that the prisoner makes between his cell and the execution chamber. The true story and the way it was scripted were certainly moving, and the subject matter was very touching. But there was something more to his words. Why was my patient so involved and engaged?

Years earlier, Guido had had to undergo emergency heart surgery due to sudden and incurable heart failure. He had told me about the fears and sense of impending death he had felt the night before the operation.

Suddenly, he had an epiphany and an intuition. And the words to express it.

Perhaps he also felt like a *dead man walking* on his way from his room to the operating theatre. He knew that part of him would surely die that day. And he did not know whether he would be reborn, thanks to his new heart, or remain forever on the operating table with his chest open. I didn't say that the nun might probably represent me as well, both patiently and affectionately attending to the condemned man in the last days of his life, listening to his secrets and final confession. In certain cases, we must try to content ourselves and take a step back.

We ended the session in silence, moved. Touched.

Both of us.

The Analyst and Giulia – Tuesday, 5.45 p.m.[1]

Towards the end of the day, the air in the office becomes dry due to the heating. I reach out my hand onto the small table that separates the two armchairs, which are identical and arranged at a 90-degree angle, so that the patient sitting opposite can choose whether to look directly at me, without straining their neck, or to look straight ahead. The same applies to me. The space between us is just over a metre: if my interlocutor and I stretch out our legs, we must be careful not to bump into each other.

After a few coughs, I decide to take one of the ginger candies on the other side of the table, so I lean forward slightly and stretch out my arm to reach the little yellow Leone box.

I make these movements slowly, without taking my eyes off Giulia, who is telling me – she only realises it now – how little she understood about her ex-boyfriend with whom she had recently broken up rather traumatically.

As I bring the candy to my mouth, I meet her gaze and notice that she is watching my movements.

The flow of her words continues steadily, the theme remains constant.

After a couple of minutes, I feel that the tickle in my throat shows no sign of going away, so I take another Leone, making almost the same movements as before. Once again, I realise that Giulia, while continuing to talk enthusiastically, is following my gestures. So, in order not to interrupt her, I point to the box, as if to say: if you want one, they're at your disposal.

"Yes, please, my throat is dry," she replies immediately.

"But how long has it been?" I ask, puzzled.

"For a while…"

I insist: "Even just now, when I first took the candy?"

Giulia seems even more perplexed: "Well, yes."

"But why didn't you ask me for them?"

"But they're yours!" she replies after a moment's hesitation.

"Mine? Excuse me, but where was the box?" Without hesitation, she points to my side of the table.

I lean slightly towards her and point out as gently as possible that the candies have always been there, on her side of the table, not mine, during this session as during all the others, in all these months.

She seems almost distrustful, as if she finds it hard to believe what I have just told her.

"If I had to testify, I would have no hesitation in pointing to your side…" she says, extremely serious.

And so, we find ourselves seemingly far from the topic she was talking about, because now there are many other issues in the foreground: Is Giulia capable of feeling a need? Of expressing it? Can she grasp what might satisfy it? In short, how can she think that the candies on her side of the table belong to the person sitting opposite her?

In this regard, my patient seems to have several implicit theories, one of which could be formulated as follows: "What I need is not available to me, it belongs to the other person, and they will not give it to me spontaneously."

This belief prevents her from seeing how things really are and exposes her to dependence on the other person, who becomes so important, as in the case of her boyfriend, that she is unable to see their flaws, limitations and negative aspects. Until she painfully comes up against them.

In fact, the digression about candies and the episode that just occurred between us helped us understand how much "selective inattention" is at work in her perceptual system.

Regaining full attention to the reality of the experience opened "the doors of perception". These doors had been previously blocked by patterns that prevented her from recognising her own needs and aspiring to satisfy them. This episode was a part of our interaction that not only described her story but also revealed the key to interpreting and understanding her behaviour.

From that moment on, it would be easier for both of us to meet in the therapeutic relationship.

Ludovico – Wednesday, 11.45 a.m.

Morning classes after waking up at dawn. Lunch at home. I was a little tired and went to take a nap. My mother woke me up. She can't stand me sleeping and wasting time. For her, studying is more than a job. I can't fail at university. It's not allowed. She's on my case like a bloodhound.

I jump up, hop on my scooter and leave. In my haste, I can't remember what time the appointment is, and I don't even check. Fifteen minutes to spare. There are two possibilities: either I'm late or I'm early. I arrive in front of the building, ring the intercom and strike a pose in front of the light that promptly comes on. Click. The door opens and I rush inside. I don't even use the lift; I walk up the four floors. I ring the doorbell and rush into the waiting room; my helmet tucked under my arm. I'm here!

I'm always somewhere between late and early. Now we'll see what happens. It won't take long to find out, just a little patience. Easily said.

In the meantime, I sit down, breathe, and my heartbeat slows down to normal. I wait.

In these minutes that slowly pass, my head fills with thoughts, vague and confused. I seem to be thinking about everything and nothing. Today, I don't even know how long it will be before I enter the room.

Time. Yes, how much time has passed? I struggle to look at my watch; I don't want to be caught scrutinising it and appearing perplexed. In fact, clocks, both real and symbolic, have never seemed to have had such decisive importance during a lifetime. The world revolves around time, and what measures it.

But time passes, and now I don't know if I was late or early. I got it completely wrong. Maybe the appointment was at a different time, maybe not even today. So, when? I'm starting to get a little agitated. What's going on? Who can explain it to me?

I immediately rule out that it could be a mistake on the doctor's part. He is always so precise, almost impeccable. Imagine, someone who always wears a suit and tie – perhaps even from Hermès – I think I've ended up with the most fashionable psychiatrist in town.

And besides, do you think someone who always has such shiny shoes could be late or make a mistake?

No, something must have happened! Maybe he's ill, lying on the table, weak or even unconscious. And now who will help him?

What if someone attacked him? Front-page headline in the local newspaper: "Psychiatrist attacked by a patient during a consultation. All the news in the crime section." He has a risky job. I wonder if my thoughts are just a bit catastrophic, even maybe slightly aggressive: could I be the patient who ended up in the news? But no, what an idea. I rule it out. Of course, I don't like waiting, and at this point, even if the appointment was only 15 minutes later, when are we ever going to begin this session?

I have many thoughts and fantasies. But few actions, so I remain glued to the sofa cushion. One thing is certain; no one can move me from here.

A few more endless, infinite minutes pass.

Until, with the usual and now familiar sequence of noises and lights, he arrives. He greets me, says something I don't register and invites me to follow him into the room. Finally. I had imagined so many ways to start the session. Instead, I find myself saying: "Excuse me, I'm not sure, but I think, I'm afraid, I'm late. I didn't know if we were supposed to meet at 11.30 a.m. or…"

"You're late? The session was at 11.45 a.m., you arrived right on time, maybe even early. It's me who's late. I apologise again."

Ah, that's what he said when he greeted me. It was an apology. I pretend not to notice and start telling the usual story of my troubled romantic relationship.

I am the victim of a kind of praying mantis, certainly in my relationship with Lorena I am completely under her spell. Even though we are far apart now, I am in fact completely dependent on her.

Last week, for example, I went to see her for a few days, obviously skipping classes, taking the train, spending a lot of money, waiting, putting up with things, taking it all in my stride. And now I feel like I'm the one who's wrong.

"Do you mind if I stop you for a moment and we try to look at the things you're telling me in light of what happened here today, between us?" When that sparkle lights up in his eyes and he blinks two or three times very quickly, it means he's about to say something important.

"OK," I say, a little surprised.

"Today you arrived on time, in fact you were early. I, on the other hand, had a problem at work and kept you waiting for a while. When I came to meet you, I apologised, of course, but it seemed to me that you didn't even seem to notice, as if you hadn't heard me. Your mind was on another planet. As soon as we entered, you started talking about your hypothetical delay. Well, I think this is a great example of how your mind works and what happens in your head when you're dealing with your emotions and needs. You had several good reasons to assert your rights – *I* was the one who was late – but instead you felt at fault – *you* were the one who was late. There may be a thousand explanations for what happened, but I would start by asking you: how do you feel *now*?

"That I have absolutely no idea whether I have the right to be here…"

"Perfect, that's the heart of the problem! You need someone to authorise you to be able to ask for and receive something. This generates the dependency that imprisons you. But the key point is that you were able to say it, and I believe that from this moment on, nothing will be the same as before. At least here, between the two of us."

The doctor didn't perform any magic tricks, but truly, since that day, coming here has been much easier and clearer. I am authorised, but above all, I feel authorised.

Now comes the fun part…

Valeria – Wednesday, 12.45 p.m.

Smile.

That's what the little picture says, a mirror that someone gave me and that I hung in my room.

Life is like a mirror: it smiles back at you if you look at it with a smile.

A smile.

That's what everyone sees on my face when they meet me.

I smile there too, in the waiting room, while I wait. A sigh.

When I hear the door close and the patient before me leaves, I sigh.

I'm happy, but I sigh. Now it's my turn.

So, I smile, I smile at him and I head towards the room.

A nice smile as soon as I enter, I look around and sit down.

But what are those pieces of paper doing on the table?

A box of tissues. That's what they are. Paper tissues in a wooden box.

Funny thing.

I wonder who has a cold.

And what other reason could justify the presence of a box of paper tissues in the study of a psychiatrist?

Oh well, it's a kind gesture. They must have been there since winter. Or maybe he has a cold. Yes, even doctors get sick. It's normal.

Anyway, there are lots of things in that room that aren't meant for me, that I don't use, that don't concern me. I'm not here to take inventory.

I start talking.

I like to talk about my life, the things that happen to me, my memories, even my dreams. I am a normal girl, like many others. Of course, I have a dream. A profession. A caring profession. No, I am not here to learn. I am here to heal myself, to take care of my wounds. They are not very deep, but they are there. I am quite sure of that. It's not that you decide to enrol in medicine – and then psychiatry – to save the world. Even megalomaniacs know, somewhere in a small part of their brain, that they are primarily trying to heal themselves. Putting on a white coat before someone else puts one on in front of you is really an old trick.

The stories that day are ordinary. I handle them with ease. I proceed quickly, without fear. We are already halfway through the session and I'm OK. Well done!

Then, suddenly, there was a shift, perhaps a turn, or rather a topic that was treated just a little too quickly. It felt like the wheels losing grip, the steering wheel slipping out of my hands, the car about to veer off the road. Bad. A bad feeling.

And unknown, because I'm a strong, steadfast person, or so I've always been told.

But unexplainably, strange feelings begin to stir behind and beyond the words. Perhaps they are called emotions. I thought they could be treated like thoughts, that you think about them, place them neatly in your head and train them like a tamer does with caged beasts. When you are sure, you can even open the cage a little. I like zoos, I would visit them every day. It is an old, almost unconfessed passion. I would even have worked in a zoo. Some are beautiful, almost perfect in their purpose: to show and control their inhabitants. You can see the ferocious beasts, but you are sure they will stay behind bars. In short, that morning I am quietly navigating my affairs, between memories, stories, thoughts, moods, when suddenly I feel a strange sensation moving inside me. Like a wave that slowly rises from my chest, up my oesophagus, neck and throat to the back of my head. It doesn't stop. At first, I thought it was a retching sensation. I knew it well. For a period during my adolescence, I had suffered from an eating disorder. They even created an acronym, DCA, to talk about it without talking about it. Because it's not right that there are people who could eat but don't, it's a real shame – with all the hunger in the world. Or even worse.

I still eat and then vomit. Or rather, I overeat and then vomit excessively. I don't like to remember that period. In fact, now I'm talking about something else. About my plans, my boyfriend, my parents, my father. Here we go, that wave is coming back, I can feel it again, what a pain. It just doesn't stop, I don't know how to deal with it, I feel overwhelmed.

My father.

It may be a coincidence, it's a coincidence, but when I talk about him, I suddenly feel myself changing.

I have always loved and admired my father viscerally. A self-made man, as they say. He and my mother gave me everything, even more than everything: education, travel, opportunities.

Here we go, the dam is about to break. That wave, still made of water and salt, begins to overflow. From my eyes, at first, slowly, almost secretly. Then stronger and stronger, it seems to come out of every corner and orifice of my face. I'm crying, there's no doubt about it, those are tears. Crying. Who would have thought it possible? That's why there are tissues, now I understand.

And here a new problem arises. How do I get them?

"May I?"

"Please," replies the doctor, pointing to the box. I gently and somewhat fearfully grab a tissue.

I carefully fold it in half, hold it in my hands and gently place it on my eyelids. The tears are also on my shirt, looking like dewdrops, or little footprints so I don't lose my way. Little Thumbelina.

I look at him. He looks at me.

In fact, he continues to look at me, following my movements with curiosity.

I don't understand what he's thinking. But I know exactly how I feel. Embarrassed.

"Excuse me…" I say, shyly tilting my head to one side.

"Why are you apologising?" The doctor seems genuinely surprised.

I am surprised in turn. To me, it's obvious. How can he not understand?

"Because crying isn't a good thing!" I say firmly.

"Oh, no?"

Silence. It's the only reaction I can muster.

I feel transported to unfamiliar territory. I try to regain my footing. To return to my own ground.

"Only weak people cry. My father always says so."

"That's an interesting theory…"

I know him a little by now. When he acts like this, he's getting ready to catch me off guard.

Here comes the attack.

"I remember an advert for a perfume. The slogan was: *For the man who never has to ask!* I always thought that message was extremely misleading and that, on the contrary, a truly strong man – or woman – can ask when he needs to. Even if it means crying."

I look at him carefully. He sounds very convincing. It seems to me that he doesn't want to convince me at all costs. He expresses his opinion, and states in a way that makes me see how he thinks. That way, I can think too.

"I can agree with that. It's true, there is strength in showing weakness. But there's still a problem. What about who must watch you cry." I try to describe it somehow, willing and curious, but without giving in.

"That's true! I'm not alone. Try to tell me what you think people who watch and witness your crying feel."

He doesn't give me even an inch of leeway. I feel him close, listening, but also hovering over me, about to make a move.

"Irritation, definitely irritation," I say with absolute certainty.

"How can you be so sure? Is that how you feel when someone cries?"

I don't know what to say, I feel confused, even a little embarrassed. I want to sink into my chair, under my chair, under the table, be somewhere else. Certainly not here.

This moment is very painful; I feel even more helpless than when I was crying. But I'm in here, in this room, and I also feel protected. I try to let my memories flow.

When I was born, I didn't cry, or so my parents told me. At least not right away. Evidently, I was trying not to bother anyone from the very beginning. It took me a long time to realise that it should be exactly the opposite. That when you come into the world, you have to cry, and by not doing so, I had frightened them. Harmony was missing from the very first moments.

As a child, I learned early on to control everything that happened, especially inside myself. My parents didn't have to spend much on nappies. It didn't take me long to understand. As soon as I realised, I needed to pee, I went to the bathroom on my own. This became a reason to be admired and a source of pride.

But at night, things changed. For many years, I suffered from enuresis – I wet the bed while I slept – and even though I tried to hide it, getting up on my own, piling the sheets in a corner, continuing to sleep in my soaked pyjamas, hoping they would dry before morning, my mother noticed anyway. My parents tried everything: more blankets or fewer blankets, more water or less water, waking me up at night, scolding or flattering me, punishing or rewarding me. Nothing worked!

One day I would understand that night-time peeing was the only way I allowed myself to cry. What I couldn't express during the day, couldn't show, especially with tears, was freely expressed at night. It was an outlet.

Fortunately, or unfortunately, no one ever understood my trick.

I would have liked to stay small; I really thought I would never grow up.

Magic.

Like a skilled illusionist, after a few years I changed my tricks.

I stopped wetting the bed at night, but I started feeling the need to pee all the time, whenever I had access to a toilet. The real problem was travelling, especially by bus, not to mention school trips. I can't count all the times I tried to avoid them, but it was always in vain, since I could never come up with an acceptable reason. I was even taken to a doctor who introduced me to a new word: polyuria. Which just means peeing too often.

No one understood, no one offered me any remedies or treatments. No one thought it could be another way of allowing myself to cry, silently and secretly. Painfully.

Other years, other tricks. We girls are very skilled at managing our flows, our fluids.

As an adult, I suffered from spotting for a long time. I believe that intermenstrual blood loss is one of the most complex, often overlooked challenges for any gynaecologist. They carry out investigations, tests, hormone levels, administer contraceptive pills with the lowest and most experimental dosages. No one asks – at least no one has ever asked me – what this dripping might express, whether it is a way of channelling and conveying other losses and other pains that cannot be communicated or shared. Later, anorexia, or rather eating disorders, were a different way of expressing my sadness, always without crying, mind you.

I really thought about dying during that period; I wanted it intensely.

"I've never told anyone this before..."

"Thank you, I see this as a gesture of trust that brings us closer together."

It took a long time to understand all this, many sessions, many words, many arguments, many denials, many explanations, but above all many tears.

It takes patience to learn to know, accept and finally love our emotions. We need to take our time, handle them with care, respect them.

Now crying no longer causes me pain. Crying is good for me.

"If we have tears at our disposal, there must be a reason," the doctor told me one day. "Since we have them, they must serve some purpose. Let's use them!"

So, I learned to do that, with a few precautions.

If I think I might cry, I try not to wear make-up. Or I go to the bathroom afterwards to fix myself up, or I use *waterproof* cosmetics.

But one thing doesn't change.

I try to keep that smile on my face, if possible. It's better to smile, at least a little. Life seems more beautiful, or at least less sad. It doesn't cost much; it's not a big effort. The difference is that now it's no longer a way to hide myself. On the contrary, I raise my head, look at the world, observe people, meet their gaze. I'm no longer afraid of what they might think. I move forward, walking confidently.

And I smile.

Note

1 Written by Gherardo Amadei and subjected to personal reworking.

5 The Cast

"Do you have children?"

The question comes up sooner or later. It's difficult to avoid answering.

At first, I hesitated for a long time before answering: I didn't have any children.

Once I became a father, it was easier to respond "yes", after trying to figure out why people asked me this question. Which in fact was easy to imagine and understand.

It came mainly from parents in difficulty. Being able to talk to someone who shares the same experience is reassuring; it makes you feel like you are on the same side.

This rarely happens now, because I'm more likely to have grandchildren. Instead, teenagers, and young patients in general, still ask me questions.

"If you were my father, what would you have done the other day when…?" one of my patients, a boy, often asked me during the course of treatment, always hoping that I would agree with his stand, but also willing to accept the viewpoint of the adult in front of him.

But his question also meant something else.

It was a call to action, within the session, involving figures other than the two of us.

In psychoanalysis, it is customary to have only two people in the room: the analyst and the patient. Other people may enter only in exceptional cases. This was also the case for me, and for a long time as well. Although my first experiences as a trainer at the university psychiatric clinic were family therapy sessions held by the professor of psychotherapy, I always felt more comfortable in a one-to-one relationship.

Over time, things have changed, and the number of chairs in the room have increased, as have the number of people. They were present in the flesh, not just in stories.

The Analyst with Carola, Maurizio, Enrica – Wednesday, 5.45 p.m.

I remember my first contact with Carola very well.

I had received an email from her requesting an appointment.

DOI: 10.4324/9781003759034-5

I replied that I was available. I also remember what happened next. Nothing.

For a few months.

Then a new contact. A phone call, strange, I must admit.

"Do you also see families? I would like to come… with my father and his wife…"

I remember it was winter, Christmas was approaching, there was no snow.

The small group arrived, but Carola was late.

I didn't know why, but it certainly annoyed the others.

"I didn't do it on purpose!"

"Of course not, Carola…" I replied. I realised it was better to be direct.

The meeting was explosive, and I later understood that this was normal for them.

A conflictual relationship, to say the least.

They all spoke about each other, intolerant, exasperated, suffering. It seemed that a lump of pain held them together, badly, preventing them from living their own separate lives. A tangle of contradictory feelings that was also played out in the room.

I quickly realised that there would be no family therapy. What I was faced with was Carola's need, her desire for everyone to get involved.

And immediately, before her departure for an Erasmus term abroad.

But doing it all together was impossible. At the same time, it was impossible to be alone, as with separating Siamese twins. So, I suggested continuing with individual sessions.

One at a time.

I started with her. It was a highly emotional meeting.

Her mother had died when she was 11, having lived for five years with one of those diseases that leave no escape. She knew it, her father knew it, and I think Carola sensed it too.

Is there a "normal" reaction to such an event? A code of conduct, an appropriate response? She had had no reaction. We call it *freezing*. An emotional "freeze" that protects us. That saves us when we encounter a bear on a mountain path.

Her encounter with the bear had been going on for almost ten years. At first, she was also sent to a psychologist. It's better than a bear. But it did not resolve the situation. Carola remained unperturbed, emotionless, living as if nothing had happened. And her attitude caused unbearable arguments and tension.

Her father became the centre of her life. Together they were everything. For at least five years, they had been each other's reason for living. But the pain that united them also blocked them. Too much love, sometimes, can hurt.

It is not necessarily true that the experience of pain makes you grow.

It must have been terrible for him too.

Secrets, hopes, pain, responsibility. Effort. Tears. Many tears.

Then her father met Enrica. Another chapter. This one was also difficult for various reasons.

And I met them too.

Two very engaging conversations. Like the others. For everyone.

When I put the pieces of the mosaic together, I saw them again as a group.

I talked about Carola's anger, a layered anger that had been building up inside her for some time.

"If I asked you to choose between sadness and anger, which state of mind would you prefer?" I asked.

The answer was easy and immediate.

"Anger!"

We all remained silent. For a long time.

Even though many years had passed since her mother's death and the pain, anger was the most effective way to process an immense sense of sadness and keep it at bay. Carola had been an understandably very grieving, very sad, suffering child. A child who had tried in her own way to deal with the loss, putting it aside, putting it to one side. Despite the help of her father and the people who had been close to her.

As I listened to her, I was reminded of the beautiful title of a famous work by Freud, *Mourning and Melancholia*. I thought that in Carola's story, the word *Anger* should be inserted in the middle between the two terms. An unrecognised emotion that began when her mother fell ill and became even more intense at her death.

It is much easier to deal with anger than sadness, because it makes us feel stronger and, in any case, alive. Sadness overwhelms us, destroys us, crushes us. Perhaps her anger was justified, but in recent years she had found no outlet for it. It is a very effective mechanism in the heat of the moment, but it cannot last long.

"And the sadness has returned…" I observed.

Again, that silence I knew so well. Almost pleasant. This time, however, it was accompanied by poignant emotions present in everyone. All four of us, I mean.

I told them about a meeting I had years ago with a young girl, a very bizarre young girl, who when she answered the phone, instead of saying "Hello!", said "Who the fuck is this?"; when she met someone, instead of "Hi", she said "What the fuck do you want?", and instead of "Goodbye", she said "Fuck off!" If the person she was talking to managed to switch on the automatic translator, they could decipher her language and the meeting took place. This was not the case with Carola, but it is likely that some of her anger should be interpreted following a similar sequence transforming pain into another feeling. This happened in Carola, but it wasn't her doing, nor was she aware of it. It had to do with the injustice that she had been submitted to in her life and with which she was constantly dealing with. An event, the loss of her mother, had not yet been adequately positioned in her heart and mind.

It was all quite clear. However, I did not know how to resolve the situation. What to suggest.

Carola took it upon herself to save the day for everyone.

"I'm the one who must sort things out, and when I've sorted them out, everything will be better. Because I realise that I have attitudes that infuriate you, I know," she said.

Again, there was silence, this time out of surprise.

"For now, we can be satisfied. This statement is very important, and I don't think she's acting or trying to make us happy."

Her father and Enrica nodded. The session ended.

After that meeting, I never saw them again.

Until surprisingly, as if in magical continuity with that last, decisive session, Carola, upon returning from Erasmus, began real therapy. Without excuses, without pretence, no ifs, no buts. Alone, she was at the forefront. She no longer needed everyone else to be there.

Life, she had finally understood, was in her hands. She was driving her own carriage. It was mainly up to her where to go and how.

For five intense years, she returned to the room, twice a week at first, then gradually less, gently.

When we said goodbye for good, it was like a new beginning.

This time forever.

Three people had arrived. Only one remained.

"Don't worry, you're in good hands, Carola," I said. "Yours!"

As is evident from this story, I continue to prefer individual relationships with my patients, and for a very simple reason: my encounter with the other person requires me to empathise and stay in touch with what the person in front of me is feeling. I admit that I find it difficult to do this with several people at the same time. So, whenever I can, I choose to stay in the room just with one person. It's my *comfort zone*, but that doesn't necessarily mean it helps others.

However, when necessary, the room fills up, together with my mind. Family members, parents, spouses, friends, teachers. Episodically or permanently. They can be families and couples, some stable, some in crisis, some reconstituted, some same sex, some traditional, some extended, some assorted. Each of them requires listening and specificity. With each one there is a specific relationship and rapport.

It is a stimulating part of my work because it requires a different way of being in the room, often with new spatial positioning, different rhythms of time, looks, facial expressions, and posture. It triggers feelings – sympathy, animosity, closeness, involvement, distance, etc. – that expose me to preferences towards one or another of my interlocutors and that alter the balance and therapeutic alliance. Furthermore, they confront me with the bitter taste of quarrelling and conflict that spills over from couples in crisis and invades me.

These are sessions that force me to deal with a different point of view, no longer that of the individual taken alone, but of the individualities that mix in the group. It is not easy…

Let us now return to the initial question: "Do you have children?"

As life and experience accumulated over the years, I often thought that it was an understandable and even legitimate question. It is not essential to have experienced suffering to deal with suffering, but it helps. In the same way, being a father has been a valuable resource in understanding how complex it is to play the roles of parent and child in life.

I then realised that the "parental" experience in the broad sense, or "educational" in the wider sense, can also be experienced in other areas. As an educator, teacher, trainer, coach or catechist.

Dealing with children and adolescents, becoming important to them, establishing a deep relationship as they grow up, allows you to receive special nourishment from this relationship that can be wonderful and rewarding. This is why it is good for a therapist who is not a parent to spend time with relatives or friends who are, to devote time and create opportunities with other people's children. If we do not have children of our own, the instructive and rewarding influences of other children in our lives can be experiences that restore the mind and spirit. It is also good for our work.

Taking off your professional hat and spending time playing with a child is a source of richness and humanity. But please beware of not replicating this scene: on a beach, a child is playing in the sand with a spade and bucket. A man, his father, a famous psychoanalyst, sits nearby under a parasol. Another man, a friend of his, approaches him and asks, "What are you doing?" Answer: "I'm watching this child playing." Watching, as if studying, not playing.

Wilfred Bion tells a similar story of failing to pay attention to his own child, so heartbreaking that he goes so far as to say, "I lost my daughter", and judged himself to be a cruel person. Except that he then became a devoted and even affectionate father, although continuously reproaching himself for the episode mentioned and for misunderstanding some of his daughter's needs.

It would be good if we played a little more and if we did it more in the room too. Play and silence, in apparent contrast, would allow for new openness and understanding.

As Roberto Benigni said in the final scene of *La voce della luna*, Fellini's last film: "Yet I believe that if there were a little more silence, if we all kept quiet for a while, perhaps we could understand something…"

6 Even Psychoanalysts Change

I had known Giorgio for a long time. He was a little younger than me, an intelligent and sensitive man. We had many interests in common and he could have been a potential friend if only we hadn't met in the consulting room. He had come to me for help with mood swings and anxiety. We had worked well together. I hadn't seen him for some time, not even for sporadic consultations. His life had been accompanied by physical illness, among other things. The first, very serious and resolved almost miraculously, even before we met. Then a more subtle, chronic illness, that needed constant observation. Now, there was a new upheaval, the future was once again put on hold, abnormal test results, check-ups, uncertainties, fears. He asked me for psychological help. More than anything else, he seemed terrified. Understandably so.

"Giorgio, you're scared shitless!"

"You're right… but you've never called me by my name in all these years…"

"That's true… and I'm sorry!"

Yes, why had I never called him by his name until then? What had prevented me from doing so? Why had I allowed myself to do so naturally at that very moment? I know very well that we must pay close attention when we change our communication style. So?

Questions that need answering.

I don't think his name came up because of his medical issues. That would have been a form of pity that Giorgio certainly didn't need and that is not in my nature.

There had been no exchanges or developments in our relationship that would have justified it.

I don't think it depended on him or anyone else.

No, it was a sign of my own process of transformation. As far as names are concerned, it began years earlier. A young patient with whom I had been working for some time suddenly decided to stop the sessions, without any explanation. I wrote her a letter inviting her to resume therapy, or at least to meet and discuss it. Her response was scathing: *How can I feel comfortable with you when your letter begins with "Dear Madam"? I need you to call me by my name… Franca!*

DOI: 10.4324/9781003759034-6

I think she was right, because in trying to get closer to her, I was pushing her away.

Since the beginning of my career, I had always addressed my interlocutors in a rather formal manner. Certainly, out of respect, but also perhaps to unconsciously emphasise differences and distances. Sometimes the desk or the couch is not enough. That's how we were taught to do it.

But fortunately, even analysts change, and I too have changed over time. Since then, whenever possible and appropriate, I call the people in the room by their first names.

And, of course, they are allowed to do the same with me.

I don't remember if I ever asked myself this question in the distant past. Neither do I remember anyone else's reflections about change in therapists. I cannot even rule out the possibility that someone may have mentioned it to me. Certainly, when we are young, we are unwilling to listen to warnings or advice about the future. We want to live in the present, and that is enough.

But at a certain point, something began to happen inside of me. Along with a new awareness.

For many years, I have struggled to read articles or listen to lectures that begin with the almost obligatory quotation from Sigmund Freud. I do not deny the past, nor do I disown the origins of things, quite the contrary. I always keep in mind a statement by Steve Jobs: "Most creative people want to express their gratitude for having been able to benefit from the work of those who came before us. Everything I have achieved is thanks to others, on whose shoulders we stand. Let us use our talents to express our deepest feelings, to express our admiration for all the contributions of those who came before us, and to add something to that journey."

A beautiful summary of the link between the necessary past and the indispensable future.

However, some psychoanalysts still have a sort of phobia of change, as if it were a betrayal. I was not immune to this, and I felt a sense of disorientation when I realised that I was changing. "This is still psychoanalysis!" I would say, almost to convince myself. I felt the need for it; I sensed the danger. Stability is reassuring.

But Freud himself – damn me, too – in 1938 quoted Johann Wolfgang von Goethe, who wrote in *Faust*: "What you have inherited from your fathers, you must reclaim if you truly want to possess it." I believe he meant here to indicate the opportunity to revisit what we have received.

Now I know, I realise, that I change every day, with every patient, almost every hour.

I wonder if they are aware of it. I feel it clearly.

Time passes for everyone.

Precisely, discovering the inevitable changes in life that stem from what could be considered disturbing problems to resolve but turn into something pleasant, a stimulus, an opportunity. And in turn give rise to research, experimentation, different ways of approaching treatment, new resources, new knowledge.

Even for a psychoanalyst, the evolutionary stages of the life cycle determine changes in the way we deal with events. Births, losses, traumas, separations, conflicts, roles, bereavements, mistakes, joys, pains, encounters and much more. Every single act of existence triggers a process that makes us different from what we were before. It is as if the craftsman within us had to constantly update himself. It is useful for everyone. Gherardo Amadei urged us to blow the dust off psychoanalysis.

Sometimes therapies themselves last almost a lifetime. What happens in these cases to us and our interlocutors? A colleague spoke about this when citing the baldness he saw becoming increasingly evident in his patients on the couch over the years. It is true, sometimes we grow old together. And with age, we must also consider our mutual feelings. Like those of old couples who know each other too well, friends who meet every week in the same bar, solid inseparable tennis, football, bridge or burraco partners, amid familiar rituals and customs.

Ending therapy, breaking up, can be difficult, just like breaking up a romantic relationship. It can be tinged with affection and habits can prevail. I have always been critical of psychotherapies that tend irremediably towards endlessness, even though I have conducted them myself. If it is true that analytical work is in fact endless, treatment should instead have an end, at least within a reasonable time frame, with some exceptions. In these cases, when there is no possibility of thinking about a conclusion, it is more necessary than ever to introduce changes, share new goals, set deadlines, and "take stock", as a good engineer would say.

Yes, it is indeed difficult to determine when an analysis is finished. We used to think that it could only end when everything had been analysed and all conflicts resolved. We talked about "healing"; I believed so and said so. Now, when I say goodbye to someone at the end of a journey, I am reasonably sure that they will be able to face life's deadlines with what they know. And that they will know how to ask for help if something or someone makes it necessary. Help that they can seek from the previous therapist or someone else. We'll see.

Sometimes, however, our patients grow up with us. We start caring for them as children or adolescents and accompany them into adulthood and even beyond. During these long journeys, we rarely think about the possibility of changing therapists, as if we were truly "good for every season". Instead, we should remember the function of post stations, which allowed travellers to change horses and postilions back in the days of carriages, to ensure efficient service and to allow animals and drivers to rest. Because, in addition to possible fatigue, we need to recognise the new person they have become in our time together. A new perspective, a new approach, a new therapist. Or the same one, if they can change a little.

Viola – Thursday, 9.45 a.m.

"Viola…" – no answer.

"Viola?" – almost a plea.

"VIOLA!" – now more of a shout than a request.

"This can't be happening! Not only have you been locked in that bathroom for at least half an hour, now you're not even answering. Do you realise we're going to be late? I don't want to bother you, you know I don't like being late, it's not polite. Do you understand, Viola?"

My father's voice reached me effortlessly through the glass of the bathroom door. I wanted to – had to – answer him, but I couldn't, I just couldn't. I was trying to get ready to go out. For me, it was hell, torture. I had to check everything, avoid, dodge, look and look again. Everything had to be in order, and I had to be clean. More than clean. Sterile. While my father was calling me, for example, my mouth was full. I wasn't eating, drinking or brushing my teeth. I was just rinsing, which was risky at that moment, so I had to be careful. I usually used disinfectants, alcohol, bi-alcohol, hydrogen peroxide, Citrosil. I had a supply, but now I was struggling with iodine tincture. Pure. Only then could I hope, or rather delude myself, that my mouth was clean, every germ defeated, vanquished. Any contamination resolved and averted. The problem was much more than just dirt.

At first, it was just my hands. I spent hours washing them. First with water, that always became hotter and hotter, then with soaps and detergents that were increasingly powerful, the kind that would guarantee to wipe out even a colony of germs in a single wash. Then I would repeat the process to be sure of the result. They say that to ensure a good wash, you should do it for as long as it takes to sing "Happy Birthday" twice. It felt like I was wishing a happy birthday to everyone in the world who was celebrating their birthday that day, every day. So, my hands became white, then cadaverous, then ruddy, and finally dry. Unpresentable. It's even impossible to greet anyone and shake hands. Shameful.

I know, my stories are too detailed. When it comes to precision, I leave no room for error, I don't miss a beat. On the other hand, it's essential to be understood. I always think that if I don't give all the information, it's impossible to understand what's happening to me. Anyway, I have a kind of scanner on my forehead. I walk into a place and zap, I see and check everything. So, everything's under control.

Going back to that day, at one point I came out of the bathroom, taking care as always not to touch the handle with my bare hand. Wrapping it in a towel seemed like a good solution at the time. And sometimes I even avoided doing that. The ideal solution would have been an automatic door. Perfect if the power of thought alone were enough, but I didn't expect that much. An elbow would have been fine too: surgeons do it before an operation and after sterilising their hands.

"A psychiatrist? Another one? I really don't think it's necessary."

I continued to beg, almost pleading with my father while we were in the car.

"Please, Dad, do me a favour, let's forget about it."

I was only 20, but I had already seen 19 psychiatrists and psychologists, I had counted them the day before. Almost one for every year of my life. I saw the first one when I was 17. Who knows, maybe it's a record.

"Ah, you just want me to look at a clinic, you haven't even made an appointment? I don't recognise you anymore, Dad. You're always so organised, nothing taken for granted. You say it's a nice place, out of town, quiet. No obligations. Really?"

"I promise!"

At least Dad was sincere about that. If he promised me something, good or bad, he would certainly keep his word. He is a man of integrity. On the other hand, I must have got my rigour from someone.

"Oh well, let's go on this trip."

A trip has never lasted so long. Years, in this case.

It's true that my father hadn't made an appointment. He had heard good things about this Swiss clinic, which was very quiet, secluded and discreet. We arrived after a long journey. He drove, I dozed, time passed slowly.

We announced ourselves at reception and after about ten minutes the doctor on duty appeared. It was a sort of surprise to find myself in front of him, not only because he was quite young, maybe ten years older than me, but also because he wasn't wearing a white coat and when he had passed by earlier with whom I imagine were his colleagues, he was laughing heartily. This didn't quite match the image I had of a psychiatrist, psychotherapist or psychoanalyst. But he made a good impression on me, he was full of life.

A few days later, I was admitted to hospital. Sure, I was not happy about it, but I really needed it.

It is difficult to reconstruct my story.

How it was possible to go from being the most wanted child in the world to a problematic, jealous, aggressive, frightened and ultimately sick child, I really don't know. But it happened.

My problem was almost immediately a fear of contact and a need for control.

Not just any fear. The fear of being contaminated paralysed my brain.

As a result, I needed and tried to control everything. To block my body.

You can have many fears in life, some are justified, others less so.

Yes, your anxieties and mechanisms are fine for you and fully justified if you're only dealing with yourself with no intrusions from the outside world. But everything gets messed up when the outside world manages to pop in and interfere, giving you advice, criticising and not understanding.

But if they don't involve the outside world, you can feel fine, somehow, motivating your anxieties and your mechanisms, and with some effort you can move within them. The problem arises when others judge them senseless, when they start telling you that this is not right, that you are exaggerating, that you must control yourself, they tell you how and what to do. And then everything gets messed up.

Sometimes it's gestures, sometimes behaviour, sometimes thoughts. It's all the same.

It is a cage in which you move with increasing difficulty and hardship. It does not matter if it's avoiding stepping on the lines on the floor, not touching objects, not eating certain food and not thinking certain thoughts. The problem is always the same. Anticipating. Everything must be anticipated, predicted, controlled.

It is as if the past, full of dark memories, generates sadness.

While the future, full of disturbing thoughts, causes anxiety.

So, I struggled to live in the present.

I didn't understand anything that was happening to me, and it wasn't as if the various psychiatrists had particularly insights. They often said strange incomprehensible things to me. One of them rattled off this sequence, sounding like a rapper: "You are afraid of sexuality, you are afraid of animals – yes, they scared me too – you are afraid of sexuality that you experience as animalistic."

Most of the time they suggested drug therapy, some suggested talking a little.

Another told me I was schizophrenic. I left his office terrified. Understandably so. Perhaps he was more frightened than I was. Like many others.

In fact, for many years I didn't tell anyone exactly what I was afraid of. I was afraid they wouldn't understand me, that they would react badly. But it's difficult to get help if you don't say what's really happening to you.

I spent a couple of months in that clinic. They were long but useful months. I wasn't bored. It was a good break.

I was looked after by the same young doctor who laughed a lot and an older one with white hair and a white moustache. He was nice and smiled a lot too: he knew how to joke around and immediately understood how to handle me. With kid gloves, of course.

I liked having the sessions in my room. The young doctor came in the evening, three times a week, his arrival coinciding with sunset, when the sun, before disappearing behind the mountains, spread its last jubilant rays and the sky turned orange. So, I would stand with my back to the window, and he would stand opposite me. That way I could see his face clearly, while he had to struggle with my face backlit. I said before that I liked to keep everything under control.

If possible, I avoided shaking his hand, and I did so for a long time, but it wasn't because I was afraid he would contaminate me.

On the contrary, I was afraid that I might contaminate him. This surprised me. It was still fear, but for the first time I was worried about someone else, fearing for his health. And, consequently, for mine. I felt that this smiling doctor had become important to me. I cared about him.

"Doctor, I understand, I agree, I need to get proper treatment. You suggested I need an analysis, I'm in. When do we start?"

"Good, Viola, I'm glad you agree with us. But now we must find a psychoanalyst who's available," he replied unexpectedly. "I'm not a psychoanalyst, not yet, I can't."

"I don't understand, what difference does it make? I feel comfortable with you!"

"Consider this scenario. Imagine you have a heart problem. It is treatable, but it requires heart surgery. I examined you, discovered the disease, and indicated how to treat it. But now you need a heart surgeon, and I am a cardiologist; I cannot operate on you. I would be crazy to do so."

Oh, blessed youth! I dug up all the obstinacy I had inside myself. I had made up my mind. He would be my therapist. I'm not sure why, but I told him the story of a stuffed animal I had, a teddy bear that I was very fond of, which I lost one day on a ferry. I talked about how desperate I felt without it. About how I hadn't wanted another one to replace it. My drama.

The doctor understood. He came to terms with not being a "DOC" psychoanalyst and we began treatment. Therapy. Or rather, psychoanalytic psychotherapy, as he told me. And as it was called at the time.

How can one recount a journey that lasted almost seven years?

It's one thing to feel comfortable, but it's another to trust, to put your life in the hands of a stranger.

I wanted that therapy and that doctor but often wanting something is not enough to make it happen.

I wanted it, I needed it. Yet it wasn't easy.

When I was discharged from the clinic, I started going to see him three times a week. The same days and times every week. Alone. I would enter the room, take my seat, strictly in front of the desk – I couldn't even touch the couch – and sometimes I would talk, sometimes I wouldn't. I would stay there for 45 minutes, then get up, walk to the door, say goodbye, never shaking hands, and so it went for seven long, challenging and sometimes pleasant years.

Consistency and repetition have never been a problem for me. I have always found security in habits and customs, a sort of guarantee of continuity. Trusting. That was hard. I was making it hard but so was he! He didn't want me. He wanted to send me to someone else.

How could I trust him? How could I risk being disappointed again?

I needed help, I was looking for a loving connection, a safe and stable gesture.

But deep down, it was precisely that contact that I feared. So much so that I was paralysed in all my relationships. Perhaps I wanted relationships so intensely that I was unable to establish any. Obviously, I was not aware of this oscillation. I remember the critical gaze I reserved for photographs of myself in my mother's or father's arms. "You see, you could easily cut me out of the photo, and nothing would change," was my comment. Contact was a family problem, I guess.

Although I was the one who insisted, going on the journey that every therapy entails with the doctor seemed impossible to me. I anticipated every possible difficulty or fear:

"If I think about it, I relive all my dramas; if I talk to you about it, you get overwhelmed and you're not the same anymore; if I hold your hand, you get contaminated too; if you tell me what to do, I'll do it; after all, it's just a job for you; and remember, you didn't want me."

The sessions were real challenges, with silent aggression at the forefront, without me recognising it. Opposing him was my first rule of behaviour.

When the doctor spoke, his words made me feel like I was facing an overbearing and controlling mother. When he didn't speak, his silences reminded me of my father, who could remain silent for days or weeks if I had done something wrong or, conversely, if I hadn't done something he expected of me.

Life is also made up of interruptions and holidays, and therapy is no exception. Breaks for me were a real drama, experienced through the fear, sometimes conviction, that something traumatic might happen to my therapist during our separation. For a long time, I spent every holiday checking the obituaries and disaster news in search of his name. It is easy to imagine how anxiously I faced those days. I often wondered how he experienced them, knowing that I spent mine waiting/fantasising/speculating/fearing that he would be the victim of accidents or misfortunes. It was enough to make me resort to spells, propitiatory rites, superstitions and amulets of all kinds. I almost gave up holidays altogether. Perhaps that was exactly what I hoped he would do.

Every now and then I wonder if it is possible to truly describe what my therapy was like, to turn it into a story, not a novel, but a story. I have already found the title: *Going through my life.* I also have a subtitle: *Contact and control.*

My pillars of Hercules.

Control. Perhaps this was the most difficult thing to change. If your head is full of fantasies – which seem real – and these fantasies are about terrible things that could happen, well, how can you not try to control everything? At least what you think you can control?

The easiest person to control was the doctor, especially during sessions.

It's not easy to go to therapy several times a week, to find the time – Dad took care of the money – or the desire, the topics, the energy In those sessions, nothing could be changed – not the arrangement of objects or the rituals at the beginning and end; the doctor's words, his interpretations, were filtered and analysed before they could even be used. It was a kind of mental hand-to-hand combat. It left me exhausted.

But I would say – once the container had been sterilised – we were also able to work and venture into the depths of my mind, my history and my emotions having managed to overcome my needy, overbearing search for the right emotional distance and my exasperated control over the other person. We were truly courageous. Both of us.

Brave and confident.

He was confident in my abilities; I was confident in him.

He confided in the power of psychoanalysis; I confided in his confidence of his own tools.

Perhaps even a little reckless.

All this rewarded us and we arrived at a conclusion that, given the circumstances, was more than satisfactory. I graduated and left for a Canadian university as a history lecturer. It was the best and most enjoyable period of my life.

No fear, no disinfectant, no crisis. Seven years had passed. We even shook hands. I felt healed. The doctor thought so too. In fact, he was especially convinced.

And then they say that we are the crazy ones, the omnipotent, perfectionists, idealists, dreamers.

Many questions remained unanswered, however.

Others would come year after year, crisis after crisis.

Why did I get sick? What happened in my head to trigger this hell?

Are you born that way or do you become that way? Is it more about genes or environment? The body or the psyche?

And again. Can you be cured?

Perhaps this is the most pertinent title for my story: *Why?*

Why did I get sick?

Why haven't I recovered completely?

For a long time, this business became our catchphrase. I couldn't accept it. After all, he was the one who made me think that everything had been resolved.

Of course, I really liked this idea. How could I be wrong?

Looking back, I think my doctor made some mistakes, to put it mildly. Perhaps he was young, perhaps psychoanalysis was also "young", despite its age. Perhaps psychoanalysis was "old", thinking it worked like a laundromat, where every stain is removed and every fear erased: "And they all lived happily ever after." Once and for all.

My experience in Canada did not last long. I stayed there for a year. I had another crisis. I asked him for help again. He referred me elsewhere. It went badly. I looked for new solutions, I found new opportunities, I asked others for help too.

I don't know why I didn't go back to him. Maybe I didn't want to ruin that memory. Or maybe, a little disappointed, I didn't want to disappoint him. Who knows, I didn't trust him anymore.

I tried almost everything available. Psychoanalysis on the couch four times a week, new drugs, lots of drugs, the fashionable psychiatrist, the one who cured everyone, a new hospitalisation, or rather two, cognitive therapy, research protocols, questionnaires, other drugs, other hospitals, other clinics, other psychiatrists, some more famous than others. Everyone had their own magic solution. I hoped for it. Everyone had their say. Perhaps the only thing I was spared was electroshock therapy! Meanwhile, I was getting worse and worse.

However, for quite some time, I didn't even think about going back to that doctor.

More than ten years had passed.

Then, out of desperation, I went back to him. I found him in Milan. His words surprised me once again.

"Viola, once again, I am very honoured that you have come to me. You have tried many treatments and have certainly not given up trying to get better. But you still haven't succeeded. Let's start from here. I have a proposal for you – it may seem strange – to do nothing "therapeutic". I believe there is another issue to work on: omnipotence. I would start with the following points: 1) notwithstanding your difficulties, you have continued to grow and progress over the years: these skills should be recognised and valued; 2) you experience a crisis when you implement changes; 3) you continue to fear letting go, but we need to find a way to reduce your control; 4) we must recognise that there are no "miracle" cures; 5) we must therefore begin to accept our limitations; and 6) we must try to set up your own "self-care". I can supervise you. I will see you from time to time. If and when you need it.

It wasn't difficult for me to accept, and not just out of desperation. I found something true in those words, something that deeply corresponded to how I felt. I had found him again.

The teddy bear had reappeared. But he wasn't the same either. I told him so.

"I'm sorry I couldn't share these things with you in the past, that we didn't experience certain emotional moments together. Now I know I'm different and that a lot depends on this different relationship with myself, but maybe… are you different too?"

I thought: if he can change, why can't I?

And so began a new, exciting phase.

We called them "servicing", like the kind you do on cars. I did my every year.

With a few overhauls, replaced parts, discoveries of new functions and modifications to the set-up.

Even with revelations on my part – you never stop getting to know yourself and letting others get to know you – that I had never imagined before. And unexpected openness and flexibility on his part. Like the time he gave me a double session – necessary for me to be able to talk about what had happened to me during that period – and gave me a "lesson" in psychiatry and psychopathology to help me understand what had happened to me. This encounter would once again significantly change my life.

Today, I am an educator, I work with children every day, I have left home, and I live with a man who loves me. I have also found a doctor who listens to me and talks to me in a new way, with a different style. I owe her a lot too. I still see the doctor. I usually go to see him a few days before Christmas. I like knowing that he is there, that he will always be there for me.

In the meantime, I take care of my passions and my problems.

Is everything perfect? Certainly not!

I have become more aware and have learned to accept my slip-ups, my unfulfilled fantasies, even the death of loved ones, my own painful physical changes, advancing age, life in short.

And I read Emily Dickinson.

7 Homosexual Archipelago

Irreverent thoughts. Uncontrolled.

Are they allowed? Why do they arise? What to do with them?

The Analyst with Luisa, Bruno, Leo – Thursday, 10.45 a.m.

I listened with sincere interest to Luisa and Bruno's stories. Parents of two teenagers, the first 15, the second 12. Two kids like many others. Problematic, sweet, rough, reactive, needy, in unpredictable and disconcerting ways. For some time during our first meeting, I didn't understand which child they had come to me about. They spoke indiscriminately about one and the other, or about themselves. A close-knit and connected family, perhaps too much so. But at a certain point, it became clear that the focus of the encounter was directed towards the boy, Leo.

"You know, Doctor," said his mother, more concerned than worried, "we don't understand why he spends all his time with this new classmate. Nothing alarms us. He's a good boy, very polite, he comes to our house, says hello when he comes in, says sorry and please, and thanks us. He even takes his shoes off in the hallway, which even my husband struggles to do!"

"No one is ever happy…" commented Bruno.

"Maybe… but to be honest, this friendship seems a little too close to me, it smacks of excessive intimacy. Even Bea, our daughter, has made comments and jokes: 'Mum, may be Leo is *gay*, it is possible, isn't it?', she said one day after walking past the bedroom where her brother and his friend had holed up, as usual."

Irreverent thoughts, indeed.

I was born shortly after the second half of the last century. I am the same age as Nanni Moretti, Pierce Brosnan and Zico, among others. Our date of birth is important; it places us in a specific time and culture. When I grew up, in Italy it was certainly not easy to be homosexual, perhaps not even to talk about it. I don't remember any doubts about my sexual orientation. The fact that different sexualities could exist, regardless of gender, never even crossed my mind. I can't guarantee that I was free from homophobic behaviour, which was certainly encouraged by the "pack", like the ones at school. I

DOI: 10.4324/9781003759034-7

remember that in secondary school I had a classmate called Eros who looked like a cherub: rather round, with a rosy, beardless face and curls on his forehead. If you add on an ever-present and redundant mother, and it is easy to imagine the "affectionate" attention he received from the class.

Later in time, towards the end of university, my future best friend and I were almost inseparable and the director of the psychiatric clinic where we were interns called us "Castor and Pollux". The homophobic allusion was clear: he considered our friendship too intimate. When that same friend of mine approached a famous psychoanalyst to begin training in analysis, he was told that he could not take him on as a patient: one of his answers had led the analyst to believe that he was homosexual. During those same years, another young psychiatrist heard these words: "I will take you on for analysis, but you should know that you will never be able to join the Italian Psychoanalytical Society because of your sexual orientation." Almost 40 years later, in 2018, the same colleague, a psychoanalyst, researcher and university professor, who is openly homosexual, received the prestigious Musatti Award from the Italian Psychoanalytical Society.

In short, the world has changed, psychoanalysis has changed. And I have changed too.

In 1969, my family decided to host an American boy named Robert as part of a cultural exchange programme. Bob spent a whole year with us. He became like an American brother to me. In 1979, he returned to Italy, to Milan, for a period of work. One evening, while we were chatting, he said to me:

"You know, Roberto, I have to tell you something…"

He had undergone his first therapy when he was still a university student, with a psychoanalyst who used reparative therapy to convince him that he was not homosexual. After discontinuing this experience, he began a second one with an analyst who helped him work on the emotions he was unable to express and on accepting his orientation. Then he met the man who is still his partner, or rather husband, because he lives in an American state where they can get married, and his marriage has lasted as long as mine with my wife. Bob's coming out was a shock for me. Among the responses I gave – some of which I am still a little ashamed of – I remember one that was embarrassing to say the least: "Um… interesting, I think it will be useful for my work."

If our brotherly friendship remained strong, it is certainly thanks to him, who was able to tolerate my words.

Fortunately, every memory is subjective. When Bob read the story about him, he wrote to me: "The response I remember, and the one I tell my friends, is that you showed an admirable level of empathy, which moved me. You immediately made me feel comfortable and normal, and I realised straight away that I had done the right thing in confiding in you. My memory of your words is unequivocal and positive."

There is no doubt that I was surprised by that unexpected confidence, but thanks to Bob, my perspective changed. Because when you see things in someone close to you, in someone you love, it becomes easier to think, reflect, get out of your own head and try to understand.

Nevertheless, our mind is difficult to govern and control. When my son was born, I was present in the delivery room. At his first powerful cry, the midwife commented: "Wow, what a beautiful soprano!"

I was very happy, but my response, albeit intended to be ironic, was less than brilliant: "Soprano? Look, if there are any developments in this direction, in a few years I'll come looking for you..."

In the same 1990s, at a scientific meeting, I heard a brilliant psychoanalyst say, in line with his colleagues 20 years previously: "If a homosexual comes to me, my job is to bring him back to heterosexuality."

It seems like a lifetime ago.

I came back to Luisa and Bruno, who were now looking at me, waiting for me to speak.

Had they noticed that my mind had wandered elsewhere? I couldn't say how long I had been consciously listening to them. They call it "freely floating attention". As always, we tend to be kind to ourselves. I would rather call it "freely floating distraction", which is more in line with what happens.

Our eyes met. I tried to be there with them, with their fantasies and fears.

"How do you feel about Bea's hypothesis being true?" I asked cautiously.

No answer.

Sometimes silence speaks louder than words. I decided to take a chance.

"Let me tell you something that happened to me. In our society – perhaps big cities are happy islands – things have changed a lot, both in everyday life and in psychoanalysis, but the problems have not been solved."

A few months earlier, I had been at dinner with a group of rather cultured, intelligent people who were sensitive to a wide range of issues in life. At one point, one of them asked me, "What are you doing these days?" "I'm reading." "What are you reading?" "I'm preparing a report on homosexuality." "But homosexuality isn't a disease, is it?" "Of course not!" I replied and explained.[1]

A moment of silence, then the next question: "Right, of course. But then, why does it happen?"

Luisa and Bruno nodded as I spoke. They seemed reassured by my sharing this anecdote. They were not alone in their difficulty in dealing with diversity. Perhaps this couple of parents were saying something to each other for the first time that they had never fully thought about before.

The possibility of a child being homosexual, even before communication or confirmation, is often not even considered. Of course, acceptance, openness and tolerance have greatly increased, but even today, coming out triggers a series of emotions and thoughts in parents, ranging from guilt ("What did I do wrong?") to disappointment, anger, a great deal of anger, legitimate concern and fear of risky or transgressive behaviour, states of threat or social shame ("OK, you've told me, now let's not talk about it anymore and above all let's not tell anyone"), genuine fears about the future of these children, about the future of generations ("I'll never become a grandmother/grandfather").

"We really don't know. We have never had any prejudice towards homosexuals, but we are not sure we are ready to consider their presence in the family..." Luisa and Bruno continued.

In some cases, I like to get help from other sources besides just my words and feelings. Books, articles and news reports can come to our rescue. Literature, art, cinema.

"I completely understand your confusion; all parents feel it when they encounter something unexpected in their educational journey. I want to tell you that there are a couple of films that could help you deal with the situation inside yourselves, one about children, *Nessuno uguale* [*No One is the Same*], and another that directly concerns you, *2 volte genitori* [*Twice Parents*]. If you want...", and I pointed to the bookcase where the DVDs were.

"Yes, we've heard about them... but perhaps it's a little early, don't you think?"

"You're right, let's not rush, let's not hurry. We're talking about a 15-year-old boy and the feelings of a 12-year-old girl..."

I realised I had been too hasty. I don't know why that story was making me lose sight of one of the commandments of my profession: patience and respect for my interlocutors' timing.

I felt some explanation was necessary.

"As you surely know, adolescents are rather turbulent. These are the years during which they begin to understand their identity, who they like, how to live their emotional relationships. Homosexuality that appears in adolescence adds complexity and delicacy. Therapy must guarantee true and authentic neutrality, but also the responsibility regarding this phase of life. Obviously, the experiences that adolescents have with people of the same sex are not a sure indicator of homosexuality, but it is also true that, almost always, awareness of a homosexual orientation is already present in pre-adolescence and may consolidate in the later stages of development. During early adolescence, emotions are experienced and feelings of pleasure are sought – *primarily* sexual ones – rather than putting yourself to the test in a relationship."

"What if this is his silent way of rebelling against us?"

"It cannot be ruled out, but Leo does not seem like a teenager struggling with conflicts and opposition, or that sees the world as an enemy."

Maybe there is no better way to rebel against your environment than declaring to be homosexual. In these cases, however, sexual orientation risks becoming a way of being, even before it has been elaborated. Perhaps young people do not explicitly ask for it, but they seem to need a hand in understanding their feelings towards themselves and the outside world. They are trying to understand whether they are facing a challenge, that of being different from the world around them, or whether it is a real internal journey. It is often very difficult to deal with these adolescents because they are the most provocative. The challenge can affect many areas of their behaviour. When it takes the form of sexuality, they become those of coitus, ergo sum.

Luisa and Bruno listened to me attentively.

"Do you think it's possible that Leo already knows and is keeping the secret to himself?"

"That's another possible hypothesis."

There are young people who have known they are homosexual for some time, but who have no idea how to communicate this to the outside world. Coming out is not a way of magically solving all the difficulties and problems faced by homosexuals. It is a necessary and appropriate point of arrival for many, but not a shortcut to solving the problem.

"Young people really need someone who can respect and keep their secret, who knows how to accompany them delicately and carefully on this journey. You, first and foremost, if this is really Leo's situation. I, if we decide to…"

"In reality, our real fear is that he may become a victim of discrimination and bullying…"

"You're right! Homosexuality combined with bullying is one of the tragedies these kids experience."

"You see, Bruno," Luisa blurted out, turning to her husband, "it's better that the doctor meets Leo!"

Often, even before recognising their own sexual orientation, these young people are harassed and humiliated, to varying degrees but always ruthlessly. Teenagers, especially when confused within the group, can be monstrously violent towards their peers. They humiliate them, and in this way try to keep their own identity together with anxieties of diversity at bay. When subjected to this harassment, however, individuals may retain an almost indelible trace of that devaluating and contemptuous judgement in their psyche. It becomes imprinted in their mind like a sentence of condemnation, which quickly becomes self-inflicted: it's right, I deserve it, it's my fault. Thus, attacked by their peers, shunned by their same-sex peers, uninterested or uninteresting to those of the opposite sex, they remain anchored in a no-man's-land, often unknown to themselves, even more so than to their parents. I also know that in some extreme cases, especially if no one notices or intervenes, death can become the only desperate way out and salvation from pain and suffering.

There are adolescents who fear diversity, for whom feeling homosexual can be a way of channelling their fear of relationships with the opposite sex. Obviously, one's own sex is much better known. As a result, closeness, contact and the possibility of being with someone of the same gender is much easier. If there is an almost phobic difficulty in relating to the opposite sex, homosexuality can become a way out, a ploy. Not to mention when being homosexual presents itself as a doubt, like a torment, a kind of panic attack. Then it never goes away. Perhaps it is "just" an obsessive doubt that goes around in one's head, like wondering whether one has left the gas tap open or closed, but with greater emotional implications. For these young people, the problem is how their thinking works in relation to every area of their existence. It presents as a doubt about sexual orientation, but it is an expression of uncertainty, a need for attention, demanding traits, perfectionist attitudes and insecurity about choices concerning many other aspects. The truth is that it is difficult to navigate these issues during adolescence.

This had been a long conversation, which began with a broad overview of them as a couple, continued with talking about their children, and finally arrived at the topic that had been occupying the mother's thoughts for some time. The reasons for a therapeutic meeting are often only implicit, but talking about them makes them clear.

"In short, if you agree, if Leo agrees, I would also like to meet him. Perhaps we will discover that it is just your imagination, who knows, but maybe Bea is right, and we just need to help him live his emotions well, as we do with everyone else."

When Leo arrived at my office, I found myself face to face with a young man who was more mature than I had expected, very self-sufficient and independent, with a marked tendency towards reflection. He was protective of his privacy and his thoughts, but open with me. It was not difficult to gain his confidence. The focus of his thoughts was Luca, the "kind" companion who frequented his home, as I knew. They had found great harmony in their interests, thoughts, moods and passions. They got on well and liked each other very much. His friend was openly homosexual. It had been easy for Leo to define his own feelings in a similar way.

"I'm homosexual, what's the problem?"

Over time, I coined two new concepts. The first was "the archipelago of homosexuals". This is what I started calling the people who gradually came to me declaring themselves as such.

Why this definition? We all know what an archipelago is: it is a group of numerous islands, so many that they may seem uncountable, or even difficult to define geographically and in detail. There is no such thing as "one" kind of homosexuality; there are homosexual people, and therefore a wide range of ways in which this identity is lived and expressed; that is, a multitude of manifestations that reminds us to consider how everyone is truly unique, in their own right.

I learned the second one in the field. Before being homosexual, Leo was "Luca-sexual".

Once, more simply, we called them "best friends". They were intense, almost exclusive relationships that began in pre-adolescence. It is impossible to say whether they were sexually oriented, but they certainly involved a great emotional investment. Then they changed over time, in many ways, often "corrected" by the rigid prevailing morality.

Now it's different. We live in more promiscuous societies, where sexual experiences are increasingly precocious, and the connection with a friend of the same sex often takes the form of a proud and premature declaration of one's sexual orientation. What happens if the orientation is not homosexual, but "Mara- or Luca-sexual"? Could it be a bit complicated to backtrack and redefine it once you have officially declared yourself homosexual? Among the many challenges it presents, adolescence also involves helping young people define themselves sexually. With respect and tolerance, but also with a critical and reflective approach. This means accepting their personal perceptions but also bringing to the fore or into the open the correct definition of the feelings and emotions involved. Freely.

There is only one request among the many that I never accept. Healing from homosexuality.

I return to my memories, to Lorenzo, a young adult.

"Doctor, I'm gay, now you have to make me heterosexual." It took a lot of effort to convince him that I did not agree with this possibility. He had also brought me extensive documentation on the subject, obviously downloaded from the internet, from Dr Google. No psychoanalyst, even a slightly credible one, thinks such "correction" is possible. It was one of the horrors of psychoanalysis, but even today, in Italy, there are groups of "Catholic" extraction that gather in the style of Alcoholics Anonymous to practise chastity: an attempt not to live out their homosexuality, in the illusory hope of becoming heterosexual.

I told Lorenzo that I did not know how to fulfil his wish, nor did I consider it feasible, but I suggested that we work together, regardless of his project. He accepted. So, we met regularly, twice a week. We were able to reconstruct his history, his traumas, and the painful discovery of his sexual orientation. Above all, it became clear that shame had always accompanied his awareness. His feeling of being different found its maximum expression in the shower at the end of the basketball games he played in. In those moments, the fear of a sudden and uncontrolled erection created a sense of panic that his "identity" would be exposed in front of everyone. Asking to be "fixed" represented the solution to all his problems. His cure.

With a sense of reciprocal trust, we agreed on a different therapeutic project which represented a truly corrective emotional experience for Lorenzo. Being himself without fear of judgement. I no longer heard him talk about reparative or conversion therapies. Nor about romantic relationships, to be honest. After about two years, our journey ended with his departure, I don't know how coincidental, to San Diego, for an ambitious university research project.

Homosexuality is a paradigm of contemporary psychoanalysis. Just as psychoanalysis has been forced to abandon a rigid theoretical apparatus, incapable of understanding and containing clinical complexity, homosexuality cannot be confined to a dogmatic definition. The archipelago is therefore an appropriate image for addressing the issue of homosexuality and the complexity of the human subject, which struggles to fit into predefined or simplistic categories. And perhaps, among the many possible metaphors, homosexuality is the most relevant metaphor or representation of diversity.

One of my teachers, Giancarlo Zapparoli, used to say: "A psychotic person can be considered cured when you are willing to give your daughter to him in marriage." Perhaps homosexuality can be considered completely accepted and integrated into our minds and our culture when we are willing to calmly accept the possibility that our son – or daughter – is homosexual and marries their partner.

As Hannah Arendt said (*The Origins of Totalitarianism*, 1948): "Tolerance is the willingness to imagine that another person may be right."

Note

1 Homosexuality is no longer considered a disease. In 1973, during discussions on the constitution of a new DSM (the manual that helps classify and understand mental illnesses), it was decided that the diagnostic category "homosexuality" should be removed. And so, it was. Then, in 1980, the World Health Organisation removed homosexuality from the list of illnesses, and in 1991, the American Psychoanalytic Association opened its training programme to officially and openly homosexual candidates. Finally, in 2019, the American Psychoanalytic Association decided to apologise to the LGBTQ community. The apology was "long overdue", according to the statement, for having pathologised non-heterosexual orientations and transgender identities throughout history.

8 Women Without Memory, Analysts Without Power

I am walking with determination along a steep mountain path. I walk alongside a person who quickly strikes up a conversation with me. We chat freely, perhaps too freely. I find him overly exuberant, which I don't like one bit. He is "too much", taking up space and making noise. He asks questions, relentlessly. Curious and never tiring. This one was inevitable.

"How long have you been doing this job?"

"Forty years…"

I think I'll have to put up with him for a long time, unless I can distance myself from him before we reach the refuge.

He persists.

"I wonder how many people you've seen… how many you've helped…"

"Well, quite a few…"

Fortunately, I find my peace and quiet again. The mountain is majestic, like its virtues, and you can always carve out a corner of solitude and peace in its vastness. I brood for a while. Then, suddenly, the last blow comes with the final twists and turns.

Promptly and precise.

"And did you cure them all?"

"No, unfortunately!" I reply. And I start to think.

It's true, I've seen many people over the years, hundreds and hundreds, the number often surprises me. I know I've been helpful to many. I remember them well.

Others I haven't helped at all, or not enough.

I remember them even better. Indelibly.

I meet young aspiring therapists. They are enthusiastic, full of energy, they believe in what they do, they invest time, a lot of time, and money, even more, to try to pursue this profession. They always ask me a barrage of questions: "How can I do this job? Nothing is happening in this psychotherapy session. Where did I go wrong? Am I really helping my patients?"

They imagine they will find a reassuring answer in me.

"Hold on to your questions, they are valuable, don't be afraid of them, on the contrary… I don't know if it's any consolation but know that I have them too even after decades of practice. It happens to me. I wish the same for you!"

DOI: 10.4324/9781003759034-8

At first, I didn't fully understand that this job requires a good dose of omnipotence. Otherwise, it would be impossible to venture down difficult paths with patients who are delusional, hallucinating, locked in their towers and fortresses. Complex.

It helps to be young, even very young, a little reckless at times.

Then comes powerlessness. It can happen after years of work, or when you least expect it. The sky clouds over, your mind becomes foggy, your brain is soaked. A struggle.

What can I do with this person? I don't understand anything. I'm not capable. A nonentity.

It is difficult to distinguish to what extent our thoughts originate from ourselves and or in what part they derive from the mood of others, the sophisticated way in which the other person makes us feel what they are feeling. It is always a feeling of even deep and desperate unease.

Feeling that we cannot cope disrupts our equilibrium and our plans.

A therapist is somehow programmed, or feels that way, to help, to treat, to heal.

Perhaps it is because of my medical training, but I find it difficult to live with a sense of helplessness. Those who ask me for help always expect a solution to their problems. I search for it diligently, rummaging through the toolbox of experience in search of a practical recipe. I find it difficult to accept that my role is only to listen.

For many, this is essential and sufficient.

And so, I return to that fortuitous walking companion, to his questions, to the many thoughts he sparked. I wanted to get rid of him quickly, but instead I am grateful to him.

I realised these feelings and emotions I have just described are part of my daily life. Sometimes they are more intense, sometimes less so.

Then some stories remain etched in my memory forever. I find myself thinking back on them with the feeling that I didn't manage to do everything I wanted to. But I couldn't, I wasn't able to.

The last time this happened to me, perhaps the most painful, was on a Sunday morning. It was early June.

The Analyst and Carlotta – Thursday, 11.45 a.m.

It's raining gently, almost warmly, as I walk along the streets that pass by the Puppet Theatre, then the San Vittore prison, and lead me to the Porta Genova Police Station. I am sad, walking nervously and restlessly.

I identify myself before I pass the guard post.

Better not to take any chances.

A short wait. A young policewoman is waiting for me in the room.

"Good morning, Doctor, welcome, thank you for being here." She is kind, affable, at ease.

"Good morning to you, Inspector. I am the one who should thank you for summoning me. I only ask one favour: you must promise me absolute confidentiality regarding the content of our conversation."

"Of course, you can count on it!"[1]

I feel like I'm in a film. Just four days earlier, I was worried because Carlotta had missed our appointment without warning me, she was always so precise, attentive and scrupulous. So respectful that she would send a text message to let me know when she was running a little late. I had decided to give her some time, knowing that she was busy with the frantic delivery of a wedding dress and the preparation of her new collection. In addition, she had recently received confirmation for a contract to dress her favourite singer. She was overjoyed. I had rarely seen her like that.

MILANESE STYLIST FOUND DEAD AT DAWN,
HANGED FROM A TREE IN PIAZZA NAPOLI.

The reason for her absence appeared the next day in the online editions of all the Milanese newspapers. I read it, but I don't understand. The name is hers, the surname too, that much is clear, but I still can't reconcile Carlotta with suicide, the beautiful, happy woman, enthusiastic about her new projects, with the rope, the tree, the lifeless body. I read it again. I am forced to believe the news, Carlotta is dead. But suicide, no. I can't believe that, not entirely, at least.

She had come to me two years earlier, immediately after her father's death, having just returned from New York where she had moved to follow her former partner, a relationship that had ended painfully in recent times.

We had started twice-weekly therapy. It hadn't been easy. She was still very attached to the therapist who had accompanied her in the past and who had deemed it appropriate to start a new course of treatment, this time with a man. The frank and transparent collaboration with my colleague had made it possible to establish trust, and Carlotta had also agreed to take medication – after lengthy negotiations and only for a short period – to combat insomnia and sadness.

She had a complicated story. She had a very intense but conflictual relationship with her mother, which she was unable to manage, despite being in her forties. She also had a sister, a few years younger than her: another highly emotional relationship yet tinged with subtle rivalry. It was not just normal jealousy of a younger sister. Giorgia had unwittingly attracted all the attention. Many years earlier, she had been involved in an accident that had made the front pages of the newspapers. Taking an ecstasy tablet had caused her acute and irreversible liver damage. Only a liver transplant had saved her and at the same time guided her in her mission: to tell her story and inform young people in schools about the dangers of synthetic drugs. Furthermore, the two sisters were born to different fathers, but the second had effectively become Carlotta's "real" father too.

Having two fathers, whether virtual or real, is challenging enough, but as if that weren't enough, another one had recently appeared, the third: was he her biological father? As usual, Carlotta did not lose heart. First, she had made it clear that only one, the second, had been her real father. Immediately afterwards, she had decided to carry out a DNA cross-check to dispel any doubts. That was her way of dealing with life. Direct, decisive, explicit. Courageous.

How else could Carlotta be described?

Free, determined, proud, an independent spirit, a woman who attracted the interest and curiosity of those she met. She seemed to have a magic touch in everything she did – and she did a lot – or in every relationship she established. She was very reserved, almost modest about her feelings, often hiding them even from her loved ones. She wore clothes she designed herself, almost always black. She was the same girl who, as a child, obsessed with order, arranged her crayons on her desk in a strict sequence of colour gradation.

With her raven hair, deep dark eyes, olive complexion, pearly white teeth and beautiful smile, she did not go unnoticed. She reminded me of Amy Winehouse. *Back to Black*. It was natural that she aroused admiration. One day a woman even stopped her not far from my office to tell her how beautiful she was. I still remember her face as she told me about the episode, her incredulous eyes, her crooked, ironic smile, as if to say, "Is she serious?"

She was a fighter, but lovable and attentive to the needs of others, even at the cost of ignoring her own.

Then Marco appeared.

He was not an easy man: he had a relationship and a daughter to maintain, as well as a restraining order obliging him to stay away from that family unit. He fell in love with Carlotta immediately. Too much so. After some initial hesitation, she let herself go. She describes the early days as a honeymoon. Passion, understanding, involvement, harmony, plans. An emotional rebirth for her.

But the bliss did not last long. After three months, the first slap came. After six, the first fight. Violent.

Carlotta ends up in hospital. The report mentions craniofacial trauma, multiple contusions, and a broken nose. There are photos to prove it: a fortnight's prognosis for her and the first complaint against him. And at this point, the first signs of amnesia appear. Or rather, Carlotta's memory becomes fragmented, disorganised; like Swiss cheese, it hides traumatic events in its holes. She knows, but she forgets. She is unaware. She does not remember.

So, trying to fill these holes becomes our common goal. While my goal became protecting her and helping her to protect herself. In these cases, it is not enough to listen, share, understand, interpret, trace back to the past, analyse the present, be a psychoanalyst, in short. We work on her mind, but also on the strategies to use to save her skin and her mental functions. Together.

She closes the door for the first time. He seeks her out, convinces her. She gives in. More violence.

She leaves a second time. He waits outside her house, effectively preventing her from leaving. They meet again. She gives in.

More beatings.

She closes the door for the third time. He rings the intercom day and night.

She turns it off. They write to each other. She gives in.

More violence, Carlotta goes to A&E again. Second report. This time Marco ends up at the police station. They hold him for a night and a day. He insults her by text message.

She ends it a fourth time. She stays with friends who live far away, in the countryside. She seems to be coping; she seems confident and determined. She confides in family and friends. She protects herself and gets protection.

If only she could remember what happened, what happened to her every time she reopened this relationship, perhaps, perhaps, she would be able to break away, to end it. But can she remember? Is this really the only problem? What happens in the mind of a woman who, although aware that she is being hurt, does not avoid it? Many hypotheses can be made.

There are people who, following traumatic events, experience dissociative phenomena, causing them to separate their awareness of their actions from their memory of them. It is as if they were watching themselves from the outside, observing what was happening as if they were a stranger. Others, similarly, are unable to connect different areas of their mind; for them, certain events simply never happened. Then there are those who have such a need for care and attention, who tolerate abandonment and separation so poorly, that they will endure almost any form of harassment rather than experience further loss. Finally, others experience emotional relationships, even the most turbulent ones, in a kind of state of physical and psychological excitement. This becomes so indispensable to them that they can no longer distinguish between good and evil, pleasure and suffering, between those who perpetrate violence and those who suffer it, between sadism and masochism.

But Carlotta lives and wants to live. She is committed. She gives it her all.

She had finally returned to Milan, to her home, when one night she was awakened by a sudden noise. When she opened her eyes, Marco was standing in front of her. He had climbed onto the roof, forced open a skylight and entered her bedroom.

Carlotta calls the police, but at the decisive moment she decides not to proceed. She is afraid, too afraid, even of losing him. Perhaps the intrusion is a sign that it is impossible to keep Marco out of her life: neither with you nor without you. Perhaps she gives up.

A month later, she is found hanging from a tree, 150 metres from her home.

Her feet are touching the ground. An unnatural position for a suicide by hanging.

The inspector listens to me carefully. She already knows many things. She herself took Carlotta's reports. But she is doing her job. She must investigate, make assumptions, find plausible explanations.

"But she was taking psychiatric drugs…" she insinuates.

"With all due respect, Inspector, if you see someone outside a bank, do you think they are about to rob it? Taking an anxiolytic or an antidepressant drug does not mean planning suicide. Would you agree?"

"So, what do you think happened last night?"

"Unfortunately, I can't say for sure – although I have an idea. What seems unlikely to me is that Carlotta could have taken her own life."

Opinions, as we know, do not constitute a verdict.

Justice will take care of that, perhaps restoring truth and honour. But certainly not life.

"*You deserve a love that sweeps away the lies*," says a verse from a beautiful poem attributed to Frida Kahlo.

In Milan, in Via De' Amicis, many different dolls hanging on the wall commemorate women who have been victims of violence. It is called the *Wall of Dolls*. From today, there will be one more.

Alba – Thursday, 1.45 p.m.

"I have no memory. I don't remember anything."

I don't know if these were the first words I said three years ago when I sat down in this chair. I don't remember.

Perhaps they weren't the first, but they were certainly the most important, the ones that struck him, the decisive ones. The ones that made me feel understood, recognised.

Now I remember very well what happened, but above all I remember how I felt.

I was crying, I was desperate, I didn't know where to turn.

The doctor even told me, after some time, that he was very worried, that he had rarely seen a person – apart from those that saw things that don't exist – that felt as bad as I did. He almost wanted to prescribe medication to me. He preferred to wait. He did the right thing.

A friend of mine, his colleague, had sent me to him. But first, I had asked him if he had ever had anything to do with my father. My father is a very important person for me, but he is also quite important in his field. No, the doctor did not know him, even though he had just dealt with a guy with the same surname, but much, much more famous.

Anyway, I don't know why I'm telling this story. Do stories begin when they start, or even before we know it? When did my treatment begin? It wasn't the first time I'd been to a psychiatrist. I'd been to one as a child, to Teresa; I'd been to one as a teenager; I'd been to one as a young adult, as they say now. And, of course, I don't remember anything that happened, not even the names of the other therapists. I only remember the reasons why I was not well. As a child, it was because I couldn't detach myself from my mother – or so I thought. When I was older, it was because of my fear of loneliness and distance (to explain this properly, I would have to tell you about that trip abroad for the school year, complete with arrival at Sydney airport and immediate purchase of a return flight ticket), then because of my problems with food and weight.

Yes. My appearance. This is a delicate subject.

I don't like myself very much. I'm quite successful with men, they generally find me pretty, but I'm never happy with myself.

Men, men. That's a rather complex topic too.

I think I should tell you what happened with them. For a long time, all I can recall is a list of rejections.

From the first one, at three years old – he liked another girl; to the one in secondary school, who followed me around everywhere, who became a monk. Fate.

I don't have great self-esteem; the appreciation and interest I receive from people is never enough for me. If I were a car, I would need at least three or four spare wheels. I always feel that the standard ones are not enough and I keep thinking that I could puncture them all. So, it's better to have spares, right?

Perhaps this is why, shortly after the sessions began, I thought that the ideal solution would be to leave Carlo. I had a therapist, no memory, too much effort to keep my life together. It was easier to "break up".

I didn't manage it, even though I tried. Perhaps that was the moment when I started to heal, when I understood that you're not strong when you run away, but when you stay, when you fight, when you face difficulties. It was very hard; a radical transformation compared to my past and my usual way of dealing with and overcoming problems. No one can imagine how many complicated situations I have run away from!

I also have two children, a girl and a boy. I thought I was an attentive and involved mother. But one day, the doctor told me that I never talked about my children. This struck me, and made me feel a little guilty, perhaps even reproached. I didn't like it! It was partly true.

I really have so many needs that sometimes I forget about the people around me.

I liked the doctor right away. I have the impression, or perhaps the hope, that he liked me too. It's very important to me, I always must be sure that I'm interesting. I can't tolerate the idea of not making an impression, of not leaving my mark.

We decided quickly to start therapy and to see each other fairly frequently. Ah, I would have gone every day if only it had been possible. Yes, why wasn't it possible? Mainly because of money. No, I don't want to blame anyone. The doctor was very kind, we agreed on a fee that was affordable for me and fair for him, that wasn't the problem.

But it is for me, in general. Another of my obsessions, in fact, concerns the idea of being poor. I'm not sure why, perhaps because my parents were wealthy but in the golden years of the revolutionary dream they donated, or perhaps it would be better to say gave away, most of their assets to the party.

But that's another story!

I really can't stand comparisons; I can't stand people I consider luckier and wealthier than me. I really feel like a poor woman.

It was one of the most important discoveries of my therapy. When I began to realise this, things changed. Do you think it's too simple? Well, try dealing with every relationship or professional situation with the conviction that you're a loser. It's not a good start, you know? It's like playing a football match when you're already two goals down!

I also played sports. Not football, but rugby. Women's rugby isn't very popular, yet we often win, while the men make a big fuss but always lose. Rugby was a great passion of my youth, perhaps one of my fortunes/salvations, because there I learned what it means to be part of a group, to be important to the team and to feel close to my teammates. During those years, I met practically all the most important friends of my life. I really enjoyed myself!

I wonder if this experience has anything to do with the issue of men.

I think it's worth saying something about my relationship with the opposite sex.

I like to be liked, and I'm not a young girl anymore, I'm almost 40. Some people call it narcissistic disorder. For me, it's always been normal. Yes, I must admit that it's an obsession or, better still, that I cannot live without seduction. If I try to do without it or if I don't succeed, I feel bad and ugly. I'm not stupid. I am perfectly aware that this creates problems in stable relationships. I know how important my partner is, how much security he has given me and still gives me. Therapy has made me understand this completely and I have no doubts about it. Carlo loves me and I love him too, very much. But I also know that all the bees buzzing around me as if I were covered with honey confirm that I just can't give up. And I also realised quite quickly that I have an extraordinary ability to like men who are a bit complicated, not to say a bit of a pain! I think it's because of the Little Match Girl syndrome I've had since I was a child.

Another thing is work. I feel like I'm pretty good at it. Nothing special, mind you. I don't have an extraordinary career, nor have I earned staggering salaries. But I manage to express my best qualities in my profession – I've always been a copywriter in a large advertising agency.

Even with my children, and now even the doctor agrees, I have become much better. I watch them, listen to them, try to understand them, to make myself understood. I adore them. I also think I have been lucky, even though I haven't won the Mary Poppins prize yet! Sometimes I just can't stand them, and I yell at them terribly. But I'm very proud of them. Deep down, I know I have a soft spot for one of them: Chiara often reminds me of certain aspects of my personality – which doesn't mean that she is my "favourite" – and Mauro still lets me "cuddle" him. What will I do when they're really grown up?

In the meantime, I've grown older too, even if I'm not particularly happy about it. I try to feel younger in every way I can. I even got a tattoo on my arm and would have gone further, with various designs, images and symbols. Then wisdom prevailed.

Meanwhile, one question keeps running through my mind. Have I changed or am I still the same?

My need to please has remained, but something very significant has happened.

At this point, I must go further…

During therapy, we began to wonder why I had no memory, what I really didn't remember. I know that in therapy you can be influenced, induced to produce false memories. But I know that the doctor didn't ask me anything nor suggest or even hypothesise anything.

One day, suddenly, after watching a television series – I love them – I seemed to remember a dream, or at least I thought it was a dream, that was the feeling I had.

But it was different.

I saw myself from the outside while it was happening. But it was happening to me. It had happened to me.

I watched the scene play out on a screen, repeated many times. Two blurred figures, broken up, fragmented.

I watched the images as if I were a spectator.

I couldn't recognise myself in the protagonist.

I was in the audience. I was detached. I felt distant from everything. At least on the surface. The absent void.

Then, slowly, everything came into focus, the characters became clear. They were a man and a little girl, and it was me. There it was, crystal clear, what I couldn't remember. There it was, precisely what was missing from my memory.

From six to ten years old. The age my daughter is now. That man was a neighbour. A person who seemed mild and kind, always available. He had earned my parents' trust, so much so that he would take care of me when there was a domestic emergency.

The ogre of the most disturbing childhood nightmares was not far away, just a few metres away, behind the next door. I don't know how it all started. Too much time has passed to try to piece it together, to ask my father and mother why no one noticed, where they were, if they had ever had any suspicions.

Instead, I know quite well why I gradually dug a deep, dark hole where I could bury that story. When the abuse began, I didn't understand any of the games that man proposed to me. I was confused, uncertain, too young to have any idea what was right or wrong.

If a child trusts an adult, they cannot imagine that they could hurt them.

At that time, I was seeing Teresa for my anxiety, and I played there too, but those were nice games. Anyway, I never talked to her about that. Shame, embarrassment, fear. I was afraid of coming across as ugly and mean. Of being punished. He was kind, everyone loved him, if there was anything wrong, I was responsible. A disaster.

Better then to erase everything, pretend nothing was happening, forget.

More so when he moved house and the games ended. Total darkness. A necessary void.

When my memory returned, when slowly, during analysis, a torch illuminated the black hole, it was like reliving a part of my childhood, understanding many things, connecting the dots. This also clarified the story with Manuel, my old boyfriend from university. He was also forgotten, erased.

"Should I talk about it? I want to banish that story, erase it, as if it had never happened," I said to the doctor one day.

"Be careful, analysis is not a magic spell…" he replied.

"Too bad. Now when I think about the past, when I remember, this thing immediately springs to mind, but then I don't know what to say. I didn't seem to have any external wounds."

"Evidently, the wounds are hidden and there are many…"

"I don't know, even when I left him, I missed him. Every time that happened, I went back. The beatings were better than the silence. Why did I return to the scene of the crime, to the torture chamber? Partly out of fear, he threatened me, he kidnapped me. It was very subtle and insidious. The same thing that happened when I was a child with the neighbour. Fear. I trembled with Manuel. When I was around other people, I was afraid they would think what he thought, I was insecure. But maybe that's an excuse, maybe he didn't do anything, maybe I stayed because I needed to. Maybe I feel bad because I must feel bad, maybe he didn't hurt me. Do you see that not remembering is a good system?"

"It also seems like a way to absolve yourself. And above all, to absolve him. As if you were the victim of a sort of Stockholm syndrome. But did you ever talk about the beatings?"

"Yes, always! We would say to each other: enough, let's put it behind us, this is the last time, it will never happen again. There was an almost mutual sense of guilt, we would talk about it immediately afterwards. Then he would start again: 'I'm sorry, but it's your fault,' he would say to me. And then he would swear, spit in my face, and hit me again."

"It seems to me that you find it very difficult to talk about it. Are you still afraid?"

"I saw so much hatred on his face."

"Did you ever fear for your life?"

"Yes! Often at night I would say to myself: tomorrow I'm not going home. He never hit me in the face, just a few slaps. Perhaps he knew how to control himself so as not to leave visible marks. If I tried to defend myself, it was worse. He would hit me in every way possible, with his hands, his feet, his mouth, he would bite me. He was a black belt in karate; he would immobilise me. I will never accept beatings again, I know that. Why am I still afraid? I'm certainly not afraid of meeting him. The problem is that when I was there, I also felt a particular excitement. It's myself that I'm afraid of. Of desiring that pleasure, of having experienced that pleasure. Violence was part of our relationship. In these cases, intelligence doesn't really count, does it? The relationship with Manuel lasted a year and a half, and it was already like that after a month. I think it really influenced all my subsequent relationships; it continues to influence me even now. The other day with Carlo, after we had argued – we were in bed – he was indifferent, and I couldn't sleep anymore, I couldn't stand it. I said to him: do something, slap me, it's better than indifference. It's not nice to live like this."

"Alba, let's go back for a moment to that little girl who thought she was playing."

There, I had already changed the subject, put the ogre aside.

If it were up to me, I would have mentioned it briefly, like a flash of lightning in the sky.

The doctor made me slow down. Relive the scene in slow motion. Slowly.

Slowly.

Details. More details. Small details.

The sensations, the moods. Where I felt them in my body. He made me relive those moments. Ruthlessly. Cruelly. Painfully.

Violent scratches on my skin. Choked screams. Motionless.

I was there, again. It's happening now. But I'm not alone.

"What could you have done differently? What would you do now? Imagine an alternative. Try it. Here it is possible."

I moved away from the ogre, at first with fear, then with anguish. Then with relief.

We went through it together. Now I am myself. Me.

The therapy continued. For years.

And today, I finally feel like I'm going to make it. In fact, from a certain point of view, I've already made it.

Another thing seems new to me. I can finally remember the things that happen to me, the stories I live. A pretty good breakthrough, I would say. Although I am very afraid that the memory of this therapy will fade with the passing of days, weeks and months.

When I mentioned this fear, the doctor suggested that we write down our memories, the story of this analysis that is coming to an end. To be honest, before we said goodbye for the holidays – before he left for that little Greek island where I'm sure he has a white house where he spends the summer – I realised that he would do it, at least I hope so. I'm not so sure I will. We'll see.

But there is something else that seems to have changed.

For some time now, I've been feeling a kind of great tenderness towards myself and my way of being and experiencing things. I can say that I almost like myself. And I liked it when I told the doctor about the concert of my favourite singer, the Boss, and convinced him to look for tickets and go and see him too. He was happy. He even thanked me.

Here we are doctor! This is a little bit of my story, our story. Which, for now, ends here.

My time is up. For me, you were a bit like one of those lighthouses in photos that are in waiting rooms. In fact, if we stick to seaside imagery, you are like a buoy to me. A timed buoy.

Like a parking ticket with coins. The ticket has expired.

And now what am I going to do without you?

Can I come back here sometimes?

Note

1 The minutes, unbeknownst to me, have become accessible, despite the commissioner's good faith. Parts of the conversation were published with Carlotta's story in *Gli uomini sono bastardi* [*Men Are Bastards*] by Carmelo Abbate, Piemme, Milan, 2018. I decided to tell the story from my point of view as well.

9 Humanly

There is a bizarre mixture of admiration and pity in this question that I am often asked:

"Why do you spend all day listening to people's problems?"

In sports, there is a fascinating concept called "*flow*". The term, coined by Croatian American psychologist Mihály Csíkszentmihályi in the early 1970s, is used in sports psychology to describe a mental state in which an athlete is so immersed in what he is doing that he experiences a sense of serenity and concentration. He is so absorbed in his activity that he "forgets" himself, what is happening around him and sometimes even the passing of time. This mental state is also defined by other expressions related to specific contexts: in some sports it is called "being on the ball", in others "being in the zone", and in the musical context it is referred to as "being in the rhythm". In my work, it promotes and at the same time derives from a good rapport between analyst and patient. It is a wonderful feeling of great well-being. It puts you at ease.

Sometimes, however, we must deal with fluctuating harmony.

You cannot be in a state of *flow* permanently. At some point, discomfort may arise. So even a person who has been pleasant and interesting up to that point – let's say likeable – becomes demanding and unpleasant. It is a micro-breakdown in the relationship, nothing dramatic. It should be interpreted as a red warning light that appears on the car dashboard: not to be ignored.

Each of us tries to do our best to function optimally, but there are moments when our human side inevitably enters the room. It is better to welcome it and deal with it.

Is it possible to meet and work with people we find "unpleasant"? Is it ethically correct to "choose" our patients? Can it be done? Do we do it? How? Can we understand it before we start?

Perhaps I should first clarify the concept of dislike and what it means to me. It is not just the opposite of liking. It is something that causes discomfort. Something rough and uncomfortable that comes between me and the other person, made up of little things, shades, facial expressions, mouth grimaces, body language, hand movements, tone of voice, choice of words. It is a more or less intense form of aversion or repulsion, mostly instinctive. It

DOI: 10.4324/9781003759034-9

arises uncontrollably, an automatism that starts in our mind and enters us, piercing and precise. We are defenceless against it, almost terrified.

I would like my colleagues, psychoanalysts, to stop calling it countertransference. It does not stem from our interlocutor, but from us. Certainly, it is activated in our relationship with the other, but it is our own doing. We should have the honesty to recognise this. Once and for all.

I confess that several times in my professional life I have had difficulty working with a certain category of men. And to think that I should know them quite well, if only for gender reasons. Brilliant professionals, people of the world, tireless workers, curious explorers of life, rich and fortunate passengers on this earthly journey, who suddenly found themselves catapulted into another dimension of life. They are dying, but they are not put up in front of death, at least not the official, certified death that we all know. It is a metaphorical end, the end of a certain way of being, perhaps an awakening inside of an existence too often taken for granted, together with the relationships and people who populated it. And then another woman shows up to be saved or who will save them. It is almost impossible for them to hold on to both their partner and this new woman who suddenly emerges from the sea of their lives, like Venus. But at the same time, it is equally impossible to let go of this unexpected gift, this sudden boost of energy.

At a surface glance, they seemingly have everything. A job, a family, a wife, children, wealth. They cannot tell us anything about their children, their wife is unfaithful, their job has no intrinsic value, their weekends are filled with multiple activities, they must read five books at a time without finishing any of them, they practise extreme sports, they seek thrills with more fervour than a teenager. Victims of a *horror vacui*, they are dissatisfied with their lives, distressed by what they have experienced, and deluded about what they will experience.

And yet, precisely because they are potentially so close, I feel that they are very far away, more so than many other strangers I meet by chance. Perhaps there is a lack of harmony because I would like them to be better men than they manage to be. But how can I help them if I view them so critically?

Personally, I have never refused a potential patient because I disliked them. Other reasons have led me to take a step back: a certain type of suffering, lack of time, life circumstances. It happens.

Then there is no doubt that I prefer to work with people I like, I cannot deny it, even though excessive sympathy must be handled with care. It is human nature, we do it all the time in our lives, work is no different. Although the gradual perception of a patient from unpleasant to pleasant is one of the many satisfactions that can be experienced in analysis. It is not just a matter of habit or forced coexistence (*every mother loves her child*), it has to do with the power of change in psychological therapy.

As with smells. Everyone has their own, and they are not always pleasant. Or with manners and behaviour, especially those that are more ingrained. They are not always appropriate or pleasant.

Managing dislike, not letting it affect you, requires a skilful balancing act. And a good dose of frankness and timing. Because sooner or later you must talk about what happens between therapist and patient and how it feels. With all the delicacy in the world, but it must be done. It's the only way that it can eventually be changed.

Most of the time, human unpleasantness also stems from a series of missed opportunities. No matter on which side of the couch we are on, if someone had recognised us for who we are, beautiful or ugly, it doesn't matter, we would know better what we induce in others. If someone had acted as a mirror for us, we would know what impression we make. If someone had told us with loving sincerity what feelings we arouse, perhaps we could have corrected something and, perhaps, we would smile a little more.

It would be nice if we could heal those who are already healed. The healthy ones.

The room can harbour many incongruities and discordance.

Let's start with the patients.

The times and spaces around which sessions and appointments are organised are the first issue.

Agreeing on therapy always requires complex and detailed work aimed at creating and defining the setting, i.e. the precise times of the sessions. So, anyone who postpones the start, abruptly interrupts, or changes their mind about the project, even though they have every right to do so, annoys me.

I am a bit "fussy", I admit. It is not my only flaw.

Yes, I must confess, I like punctuality in meetings, neither early nor late. At the same time, having carefully designed a waiting room means that it has become a pleasant place to stay, even for a long time, sometimes a very long time.

Then there are also delays, which can actually be convenient, or absences, which can be even more convenient.

Patients who habitually arrive after the start of the session may come across as uninterested, sloppy or disrespectful, but worse still, it can induce in us a sort of tacit and collusive harmony with his disharmony. It is so convenient to have few moments to switch off, read emails, stretch our legs, open the window, reply to WhatsApp messages, air the office, eat a chocolate, make a phone call. It may even happen that we can appreciate this patient, despite the potential hostility in their delay. They are giving us their time, so why change anything? It is a tempting thought.

I also like stability: once a day and with the time set, I would like it to remain that way forever, except in very rare and well-justified cases. But I try to commit myself to adapt, and as soon as I can, I accommodate those who ask me to reschedule or make up for a missed session.

On the other hand, I cannot stand those who make an appointment and cancel it at the last minute, or do not show up and do not even notify me. Especially those who schedule a first meeting and then disappear. Over time, I have developed a sort of personal rant that I unleash on the unfortunate person, if I can. It consists of three points:

- They have shown a lack of respect for me. This job also allows me to make a living.
- They have shown a lack of respect for themselves. Continuity is necessary for therapy to be effective.
- They have shown a lack of respect for others. especially the people who couldn't get the appointment they need.

Not to mention those who do not pay for the services they receive and disappear into thin air. On a few occasions, after repeated and futile attempts to recover the debt, I invited the debtor, if they really did not want to pay, to donate the missing amount to charity. I have no evidence whatsoever that anyone has done so. But I like the proposal, the nature of the gesture.

Then there are those who leave their plastic cup or empty bottle on the table before leaving; those who leave a used tissue behind; those who fill the office with scattered personal items, such as a phone on charge that rings incessantly, so you must get up to check it every time. Those who always arrive significantly late but call you from their car and want to start the session on the phone so as not to lose "their" therapy minutes. I could give many other examples, but they are always about a lack of consideration.

I cannot really come to terms with disinterest in others because it is so inconceivable and painful for me. So, I gradually update a personal and secret *blacklist* in which I keep track of missed appointments or payments. Some would call it "business risk". I need it in dark and difficult moments to remind me how much effort my work takes and how legitimate it is for me to charge what is fair to do it (to each person according to their means, to each according to their needs).

We are not the only ones who observe. Patients scrutinise us too.

"I've noticed that at times you wring your hands and bite your nails a little… is that right?"

I am also grateful to those who furnish me with less pleasant images of my presence in the room.

The days in the office, whether long or short, leave their mark on us. The forced posture, the lack of movement, constant listening to other people's stories, all leave traces. It is inevitable that boredom, distraction and an apparent lack of attention may appear at times. Some signs of nervousness and impatience. Even the drowsiness that Adele will have to deal with shortly. This job can become a routine which is difficult to break, impossible to get rid of, hardly likely to be contrasted with massive doses of coffee or dietary measures during the lunch break. There are just moments and people with whom this happens. That's all there is to it.

We should not be afraid or ashamed of all these less than functional aspects. If anything, it is important to be aware of them, to accept even the less noble and flattering moments.

This, ultimately, is the answer to the initial question: I can spend all day listening to people, primarily because I enjoy it and am interested in it, but also because at times I allow myself to feel tired, bored, displeasure, some anger, even fear and discouragement and more.

The normal states of mind of any human being. I reread these pages and can identify myself in them, perhaps too much so.

During the long process of writing this book, I often wondered whether it was necessary to write it, to put so much of myself into it. Those who accompanied me on this adventure pushed me with gentle determination. Those closest to me always expressed their doubts. Some even advised me to sign it with a pseudonym. Instead, I put my face to it.

And now, after everything I've said, and what's to come, I also feel like there no walls around me, and perhaps no clothes on me. Or better yet no safety net.

Adele – Thursday, 2.45 p.m.

I don't know why, but Giorgio Gaber's song "L'elastico" ["Rubber Band"] comes to mind. It talks about someone lying on a couch surrounded by silence. And of a tape recorder starting up.

Our room that day was not silent at all. I talked and talked, told stories and more stories, perhaps always the same things, even a little boring. Work, family, love affairs. Just one. The only one I really wanted. In the meantime, I was content with the attention of an older gentleman.

Today I think it was a sort of reversed transference, whereby I made do with the little and questionable love I received from this man, since I couldn't have it from my analyst.

The fact is that I talked about this relationship all the time. Perhaps I was also hoping to make him a little jealous.

I'm not exactly a beauty, but I am pretty, with brown eyes, long blonde hair, perhaps a few pounds more than necessary, but well distributed over a harmonious figure.

However, seducing him was out of the question. He was inflexible.

Strict. Incorruptible.

Fuck off…!

I talked and talked.

It was my, our way of being in that room. Dreams, hopes, disappointments, work, projects, my little and big world.

My family, my hard work.

I loved my father very much, a successful, well-known and respected man. I think I always chased after him, hoping for his attention, for a "special" look, different, just for me. In vain: he was always too preoccupied with himself.

Work came first. Then photography, friends, a stormy relationship with my mother.

And after the separation, as I had predicted, things got even worse. His new wife and son, my brother were at the top of his list of priorities. A boy. I don't know if a sister would have been better or worse, perhaps a tragedy either way. A boy, however, sounds like an heir: the lineage continues, the surname is passed on. At that point, I lost every chance. But I was stubborn. I still am. For better or for worse.

In all the things I can have, but even more so when they are impossible. So, despite the evidence, I continued to hope that the situation would change, that finally I would get some attention all to myself. Even if it was just a phone call.

"Hello! What are you doing today? How about going out for lunch together or going for a walk?"

I'm not talking about going shopping or accompanying me to a concert. Just spending some time together, the two of us, without feeling like it was time stolen from his life, or worse yet, a secret. Secrets are beautiful if they make you feel unique, special, "just the two of us in the world, in our souls". But not when they become clandestine, subterfuge, guilt. Oops…

Is anyone thinking that the aspiring lover, who was older and clandestine, had something to do with my father?!?

To be honest, I must say that I didn't miss out on any loving figures.

My mother, we fought so much, my grandmother, my beloved granny. I found her when she left us forever. But for a girl, a girl like me, a little fragile and uncertain, a father, a man, is something else. Now things are better, but deep down I still haven't come to terms with why it happened.

Anyway, let's go back to that room, to that day. I don't think I'll ever forget it.

I talked and talked.

The doctor was silent. That was never a problem for me. It's called analytical listening, I know it well, it doesn't mean distraction or disinterest. Now they call it mindful attention. It's a participatory and reassuring silence. It's nice to be listened to, it makes you feel good, it makes you feel a little special. Someone who is there, paid, just for you, no one else in the room, no phone calls, a few parcels arriving, but not all the time, someone who is there when he is there. Precisely, when he is there.

Because he remained silent, but not too silent. Not silent. Not totally silent. And at a certain point, the silence began to become thick: I could hear his breathing, which is a good thing, at least it means he's alive, it's reassuring. But that breathing was becoming too rhythmic, too intense – how can I put it? – increasingly "breathless".

I stopped talking.

It happens; it had happened before.

Usually, especially if I interrupted the story abruptly, after a few moments his voice would appear, curious, interested. Confirmation that he was there and listening to me.

"Has something happened?"

And from there, the conversation would start again. Not that day.

I was silent, he was silent. And "breathless".

After waiting a while, at least I was sure he was alive, I overcame my hesitation and took the plunge.

"Doctor…" Nothing.

"Doctor?" Still nothing.

"DOCTOR!"

Well, maybe I didn't shout, even though it felt like I had let out a primal scream.

His breathing returned to normal, there were small noises, some movement, the sensation of a body coming back to life and assuming a more comfortable position.

He cleared his throat: "Yes… tell me…"

I would have really loved to reply, like when I was at school: "Now, tell me, what was I saying? What were we talking about? Pick up from the last sentence!" Instead, I remained silent. What should I say to him? How do I get out of this mess? Can I ask him what I want to know? But then, do I really want to know? Ugh, my usual insecurities.

When in doubt, I continued to remain silent.

There are situations in which the best choice, the "least wrong" one, is to remain silent.

Silence. Silence. Silence.

"What's going on?"

The question reassured me a little. I had found the doctor I knew. But the problem was not at all resolved. Now more than ever, it was up to me to speak. Yes, speak. To say what? The more that question ran through my head, the more I thought I had made a mistake, that I should have kept quiet, that I should have left him alone. I could have kept talking, it didn't matter that he wasn't listening to me, that he was… I could have avoided this terrible moment. But now I was in too deep, I couldn't play the silent game, he would have won anyway.

So, I threw myself into it. I don't even know how.

"I need to tell you something. I need to ask you a question. But I'm afraid to ask it. How can I say it?"

Silence again.

"Using the Italian language…"

Now he's being funny too. Is he serious or is he pretending? More silence.

"And then, will you answer me? Although I don't know if I really want you to answer me!"

"Let's see. If I can answer your question, if you really want me to, I'll be happy to."

There it is again, his reassuring tone, the one he uses on important occasions, the one that keeps me here. It's his job, it's his job. But it works.

And suddenly, courage. All at once. Doubt.

"But were you asleep, Doctor?" Silence, silence again.

And waiting.

Now he's getting angry, really angry. He's going to send me away, I know he will send me away, he doesn't want to see me anymore, but what have I done! I should have stayed in my place, kept talking about my business, who cares what he was doing.

Waiting. Anxious this time. He starts talking again.

"You see, Adele, it would be very simple if I answer yes or no. With all the consequences that would entail. But there is only one way to kill a question: to answer it. And perhaps we would miss an opportunity. Your question is very important, it is precious. It touches on a key aspect of our relationship. It speaks of us, of me, of my presence or absence. It seems crucial to me. So, I'll make a proposal to you. I promise that I will answer in the end, if you still want me to and if it is necessary, but in the meantime, I suggest we work on what happened between us, and especially within you. How you felt, what you experienced."

I accepted, not for the sake of peace, but because I sensed something genuine and sincere in his words. He didn't want to run away from his responsibilities. He could have taken refuge in interpretations (you're telling me that… your experience is that… you feel like someone who…), passed the buck to me (you heard that…), remained silent, which always wins, hid (I wasn't sleeping, I was having visions about the two of us. It happens to me often…). Instead, I felt he was putting himself on the line, without protective barriers, and at the same time trying to protect me.

"Good! Can you tell me what happened before?"

I'll explain, starting with what I was saying, about his silence and my feeling that he was "too" quiet…

"Good, I'd say that's clear. Now we have two possibilities. Either you had the right feeling, *that I actually dozed off*, or you were wrong, *that I was quieter than usual*. You have 'your' truth, which you are quite convinced of. But let's start with the second hypothesis, the misperception. According to this hypothesis, how did you feel, how do you feel now?"

"That it was all my imagination. That I was boring and repetitive. And I attributed my own feelings to you. You call it projection, don't you?"

"It gives me a great escape route! All right, let's keep it there…"

He didn't even let me reply.

"Let's say, instead, that your feelings were correct, that I was actually asleep. How did you feel? What did you think?"

"If you really were asleep, it means I'm a piece of shit."

"Actually, if I really was asleep, it means I'm a piece of shit!"

Another silence. And awkwardness.

"What else did you feel?"

"That you couldn't stand my repetitive talk and my unchanging behaviour anymore."

"So, you didn't think I was the one who was out of place, inattentive, bored. Is it so impossible to get angry with me? Is it easier for you to always take responsibility for the things that don't work?"

"Perhaps for a moment I felt humiliated, it was terrible, and it was even more terrible that you were the one who made me feel that way, but then I decided that I had to save you, that if I saved you, I would also save myself. So, I took all the blame."

"But look what's happening to you here! For a moment, you were convinced that I, your therapist, the one you go to and pay to help you, had fallen asleep. For a thousand possible reasons, even the most human and understandable ones. But still asleep! Whether right or wrong, you were convinced. I think it's an extremely unpleasant feeling, which can give rise to a wide range of varying emotions. Pain, anger, sadness, abandonment. Everything is silenced by the conviction that you are boring. How do you explain it?"

"So that I don't lose you. Or at least I don't lose the image I have of you."

Like a child who is scolded and thinks that at least his mother cares about him, or a woman who is beaten and thinks that at least a hand has touched her body.

He was right, it's called "attention seeking".

Little, almost nothing, even if it is ugly and unpleasant, is always better than absolute nothingness, indifference. The perpetrators know this well: this is how they manage to obtain the complicity and silence of their victims.

I too was suffering in this situation that had just happened during the session, but once again I confirmed my position as the "victim" and saved my "perpetrator". Now it was clear to me, I had experienced it first-hand.

People often ask me to describe what therapy is, what really happens, what makes it so special. It is almost impossible to explain. My analysis lasted over many sessions and a long period of time, months, years. Not every session was memorable, but the turning points always coincided with those moments when I felt we were deeply "in sync"; when I could describe our therapeutic relationship as an *encounter*. They are called "present moments". I don't know how many there were, I never counted them. But there were enough.

The analysis then continued and ended, albeit temporarily, as often happens. Every now and then I returned to my analyst to deal with certain stages of life. We meet face to face now, no couch. And I always feel awake. In fact, sometimes I am the one who arrives tired, sleepy, exhausted. And when I leave, I feel more energetic and alive.

Even psychoanalysts change during and because of therapy.

Right, Dr Sleepyhead?

10 Houston, We Had a Problem

"I certainly don't mean to lecture you on your job, but I think you've made a few mistakes yourself… Are you sure you never make mistakes?"

Discord

A good meeting stems from good rapport. This is not always possible.

I remember when a colleague sent me a 40-year-old woman, Lucia, to start therapy. In fact, he had given her three different names – I don't like this type of procedure – to choose the one she thought best suited her needs. We had a satisfactory first meeting and made a second appointment to get to know each other better. That meeting never took place.

"Doctor, I have decided to go elsewhere, to another colleague who was recommended to me. It's nothing personal; I liked you. I had some issues with your waiting room: it looks like a real estate agency. I wouldn't feel comfortable there."

This was the reason I received a few days later.

Had I been too kind? Too welcoming? Too much attention to the studio? Too many candies, perhaps.

I hope that the waiting room she chose, the next property she "rented", was able to put her at ease. I like to think so. I really hope so.

Mistakes due to inexperience

I'm going to be upfront about this, I know.

I was quite young, both in terms of age and profession. An ambitious aspiring psychoanalyst, I was looking for a "case" to begin my first certified analysis for training. For those who don't know, every "candidate", i.e. an analyst in training, must conduct at least two therapies under the clinical supervision of a supervisor. I had succeeded thanks to a colleague who had sent me a patient willing to undergo therapy with several sessions weekly.

I was, therefore, delighted. But greedy. How can I put it? One bar of chocolate wasn't enough for me; I wanted another one. Mine. Only mine.

The new request that had arrived spontaneously at my office seemed perfect.

DOI: 10.4324/9781003759034-10

Maria, a woman, suffering but not severely. A secure job, financially independent, with relationship issues on the emotional side, interested in psychology, aware of the rules of therapy and the possible results – a friend of hers often told her about the good analytical experience she was having – willing to start a course of treatment. What more could I ask for?

Exactly.

At the first interview, I suggested to start immediately, the following week, with four sessions of psychoanalysis a week, on the couch. She accepted immediately. I felt like a fully-fledged psychoanalyst.

On Monday of the first week, the patient arrived punctually for her appointment, entered the waiting room, came into the office at my invitation, went to the couch, sat down and began… to remain silent, mute, inert.

I felt surprised, bewildered, disoriented. I tried in every way to understand her reasons, to break the deadlock, with words, my own, with sympathetic and welcoming silence. Nothing.

The psychoanalysis lasted for the four sessions of the first week. That was all.

The following Monday, she did not show up for the session and informed me of her decision to discontinue therapy. I never saw her again.

What I mean is that in our work it is rather important to understand whose needs we are dealing with, ours or those of our interlocutors. Confusion can usually cause a big mess.

In the story I just told, I don't know if it was worse to suggest therapy at the first meeting, without even giving us time to get to know each other a little and understand what would be useful for her, or to "impose" the four sessions. Perhaps both: haste and greed. An explosive mixture.

At the time, I didn't fully understand how much it costs to devote time to one's own care.

I understood it very well when I realised that, for another patient who came from a distant city, the single weekly session required the time of a four-session analysis.

Some time ago, a colleague told me that when she was young and eager to help, she had suggested three or four sessions a week to a new patient she had just met.

"I don't know, Doctor… three, four… that's fine…" was the reply. "But I was thinking of doing a few more, I don't know, five, even ten. Yes, I could do about ten sessions!"

In all.

Money, money

"Good morning, Doctor, my GP gave me your name. I'd like to make an appointment. But can you tell me how much a consultation costs?"

I don't like giving this kind of information by email or text message, or even over the phone.

I understand how important money is for people, how important it is in our work, the enormous commitment people take on when deciding to undertake therapy, especially when it can be long and often unpredictable in duration, such as analytical therapy.

I also understand the need to know exactly how much a visit will cost in advance. Everyone has the right to understand whether they can afford treatment. Even just to know the cost.

However, as far as possible, I try to postpone financial matters until the meeting, when we can look each other in the eye and find a solution *that is good enough* for both of us. Although it is not always possible or right to postpone.

In general, it is easier to imagine that psychological therapy cannot begin or be carried out because of its cost, unable to bridge the gap between the therapist's demands and the patient's resources. In my experience, this is not the only reason. And often it is the opposite.

I remember having an excellent meeting with Franco, a young lawyer. He was talented, intelligent, studious, had a brilliant university career, passed his bar exam on the first attempt, and was adequately ambitious and determined. His first job in a large and prestigious law firm left him little time for his loved ones and his passions. He suffered from this but was unable to find a solution. Panic attacks and a subtle sadness undermined his quality of life.

He asked for help, he knew he needed it, he had faith in psychotherapy.

We had never discussed money during our sessions. At the end of the first session, he left without paying, without even asking if he owed me anything or how much. I had remained silent, undoubtedly colluding with his blind and silent area. I enjoyed working with him, perhaps fearing that I would ruin the atmosphere of understanding and alliance, that I would rock the boat. When it came time to share and decide on the start of therapy, the issue could no longer be postponed. When he asked "how much", I made him my proposal.

"That's too much," he replied. "I can't do it." I reacted as I usually do.

"I understand. Let's do this. Tell me what a possible amount for you is and we'll see."

He made a reasonable offer which I accepted. It had been a quick negotiation. He seemed very satisfied.

He expressed his satisfaction with the agreement. He showed sincere gratitude, and we set a time and day for our meetings. Everything seemed fine.

To my surprise, soon after the lawyer cancelled our appointment and informed me that he wanted to suspend of our project, adding, for now. It never resumed.

We always need to understand and explain the reasons behind the events that affect us; it is part of our DNA. We thrive on reasons and explanations.

In this case, I have reasonable grounds to believe that postponing the mediation of the fee and its quick resolution, thereafter, combined with my initial discomfort regarding the matter, left room for fantasies – or ghosts – that compromised and finally impeded our work together.

Apparently, it is impossible to separate what may be beautiful and fascinating, ideal and noble, ethical and philosophical, but also very concrete and practical from seemingly prosaic issues such as money. Even if there are those who try.

Parents against

"Good morning, Doctor. I confirm that my daughter will be discontinuing therapy after the next session. I don't want to argue, but I want to be clear. Let's get to the point. Sonia has not shown the slightest improvement. Obviously, I am referring to the Sonia who lives with us. The only one I can interpret. I am not a psychologist or a psychiatrist, but a mother. I am not judging, mind you, but interpreting the signals, all negative, that my daughter sends me. I am careful not to express an opinion about you or the therapy you have implemented. I am simply telling you that in recent months you have gained a patient. I, on the other hand, have lost a daughter."

After a long and exhausting confrontation with Sonia's parents, we had reached the dreaded conclusion. A unilateral and irrevocable decision. Stop. There were no alternatives. Unfortunately.

Yes, I am quite familiar with the problem, having dedicated myself fully to hypotheses, theories and supporting evidence 360 degrees: in therapy with adolescents, you must find a place for the parents and establish a good relationship with them.

In practice, this theorem is much more difficult to apply.

I know very well that entrusting a child to a stranger – even if they are a psychotherapist – can cause a range of feelings: pain, a sense of failure, worry, humiliation, anxiety.

We spend our lives warning our children – don't take candies from strangers – and then we leave them alone in a room with someone we barely know.

In my early years as a young therapist, I struggled with parents because I liked their children too much and was biased in favour of them. Once I grew up and became a father myself, I found myself to be less critical and harsh and developed greater understanding towards parental figures. Nevertheless, clashes with some parents, especially mothers, still occur from time to time. It seems inevitable, practically hopeless, alas.

What are my responsibilities, what are my shortcomings?

I ask myself if I have always remembered their efforts? Have I truly thanked them for the trust they placed in me? Have I asked them for their help and cooperation to join forces in the delicate responsibility of supporting their children in the process of growing up? Have I felt real gratitude and respect for allowing me to work with their children?

Again. When a child spoke badly of his parents, did I remember that only he is allowed to do so, while I am not allowed to do so in any way?

Someone said: let he who is without sin cast the first stone. How can I disagree?

There is no room for me

For some time, I had been treating Stefania, a young adult who was suffering greatly. She had a history of deviant behaviour, including substance abuse and emotional and relationship problems. I had managed to gain her trust. She came to the sessions regularly trying to put a new order in her life. She felt she could do it, and she was committed, despite the effort it took.

That morning, I went to meet her in the waiting room as usual and greeted her, but she did not budge from where she was sitting. Surprised by her reaction, only a moment later I noticed there were two other people in the room, a man and a woman.

After a moment's hesitation, she pointed them out to me with a nod of her head: "Aren't they supposed to come in?"

Now I recognised them.

"They" were two celebrities, well known in the gossip columns because of their ongoing separation. In fact, they were undergoing family mediation, and they had an appointment with my colleague who works in the same office of mine.

"No, it's your turn. I'm waiting for you," I said curtly. The patient slowly left the waiting room, but not before greeting the woman and telling her how beautiful she was with enormous admiration.

"I thought they had the priority," she had reiterated as soon as she entered the office.

At the end of the session, she said goodbye to me: "This isn't my place, I can't come here if these important people come."

It was impossible to find a remedy to undo what that experience caused her to feel. Perhaps her desire to feel like a star was overwhelming. But then again, maybe I failed to make her feel that she was important for me. Perhaps we had not yet worked on the feelings of shame and inadequacy that her personal history had left in her.

I had lost a patient. She had given up an opportunity.

To be continued

I am sorry for the mistakes I made. For what I did not understand.

For what I will never understand.

11 Red Lights

There are many legends about romantic escapades in the room. Not to mention the sexual ones.

How did they come about? How did they spread?

How much of it is true?

There is no doubt that there can be no cure without emotional involvement.

A universal truth? However…

Winter, late afternoon on Sunday. On duty at the clinic. Almost evening.

There is a sense of emptiness, an inertia that slowly descends like a veil over my mind. Loneliness. A sort of lazy languor. Like some Sunday afternoons of my childhood, spent between lunch, a nap, *football commentary*, a book and boredom. So much boredom.

Luckily, there is a television here. A good pastime, I think, when the telephone rings in my room, the doctor on call's room.

It's the nurse on duty.

"The lady in room number 12 would like to talk to you. Is that possible?"

I arrange to meet her in a doctor's office. In hindsight, it seems like foresight.

She joins me a few minutes later.

Introductions, quick pleasantries, and she immediately starts talking. Small problems, no drama, a few jokes. I wonder if she was bored too.

In fact, Sundays at the clinic must be long and unending for everyone.

Perhaps it's an excuse. What's really going through her mind?

What does she want?

I get distracted. I follow my thoughts.

Rumours have it that many years ago, in the office just opposite this one, a young colleague ended his first consultation with an attractive patient with the following words: "I can refer you to a colleague of mine for your problems. As for the two of us, how about going out together tonight?"

Romantic relationships, flings and marriages have also blossomed here. Could there be strange influences at play? What kind of relationships can develop between psychiatrist and patient?

I return to my late Sunday afternoon company.

DOI: 10.4324/9781003759034-11

She is beautiful, elegant, sweet and austere. Suffering.

Fascinating. She knows it.

Once again, I lose myself in my thoughts, distracted by her irrelevant words.

In an instant, I find her next to me, she has crossed the protective barrier offered by the desk. I feel a sense of threat; there are no more boundaries. Suddenly our positions are unequal, I feel the need to jump up out of my chair almost as if she had created an animalistic challenge. I jump up, try to move to the side, but in a flash, I am with my back against the wall and suddenly she right in front of me. No escape.

Before I even see it, I feel her face approaching mine, like an air-to-air missile with a laser pointer. Instinctively, I turn my face away. I don't know where I learned this, it's the first time it's happened to me, but it works perfectly. Her mouth misses, her lips touch the air, her tongue already out, wetting the wind. At this point, I raise my arms to push her away, my hands are on her, I touch her.

I shouldn't. You mustn't.

She insists, determined, fearless, shameless.

Without knowing how, her hands now are on me, quick, skilful, precise.

My belt is undone, my trousers too. She looks like the goddess Kali. How many hands does she have?

I overcome the shock and surprise, gently pushing her away. Gently.

She is still a woman, even if she has the strength of a bulldozer.

She is a patient at the clinic; I am a doctor.

She seems to accept it, stops, walks away, she understands, thankfully. Reasonable. That's fine.

Then, unexpectedly, even more so than before, another sudden movement.

Her lips are now on mine, her tongue in my mouth.

What do kisses taste like?

This time I don't stop, I don't stop her. We end up on the floor, on a carpet that I wouldn't want in any house now, but which seemed so elegant, welcoming and cosy at the time.

One question, one scruple. If she were less beautiful and charming, would I still be here with her?

We'll think about that later, if necessary.

We are already lying down, I feel her desire, I am about to give in to mine when a terrifying thought flashes through my mind: could she be armed? What if she has a razor? In those years, Lorena Bobbit, the American woman who castrated her husband, was every man's nightmare. No, her plans seem to be something else, and at that moment they coincide with mine. She is hot, and so I am.

I want her. "No risks?" "No, I stopped, you know how it is…" Fear. Not of disease, I'm a doctor, I don't get sick. But of a child. No, not that, it's a bit early, I'm not ready. In an instant, I pull away, I'm out of danger. Safe.

There are many ways to have sex, you know that too, it doesn't surprise me. In an instant, plan B kicks in. Another bizarre thought – why is it that stupid news stories always stick in my mind? – leads me to Monica Lewinsky. I think I'm getting carried away, I'm not in the Oval Office. It's true that the clinic is in my hands right now, but I'm just the doctor on call.

Yes. I'm in danger. What am I risking?

Madness, being discovered, tomorrow, a complaint, the Medical Council, being struck off.

The fantasies? Even bigger. We will love each other, I will marry her, I will know how to cure her, she is rich, we will live an eternal holiday: illness stems from pain and lack of care, but I will be her doctor. It will be wonderful, like this moment. Which is fantastic. She does it, and she knows how to do it. She is good, quick, essential, because she wants me, she wanted me. And I want her too. Who cares what might happen, let's just go with it. Come on.

I can already hear the nurse's footsteps approaching, she must take the patient back to her room. I imagine the hand knocking discreetly, the door opening silently, the horrified look that falls on us.

And finally, I open my eyes.

In psychoanalysis, we call it *rêverie*, but we could also call it fantasy or imagination.

How many events can be contained in a millisecond, an infinitesimal fraction of time? How far can we push our minds into that parallel reality?

A series of highly emotional events are unfolding in the room that has seen so much and continues seeing more. Many involving both of its inhabitants.

After all, those two, the two of us, are nothing more than human beings who recklessly and dangerously enter an intimate, exclusive and profound relationship, difficult to clearly distinguish from a romantic relationship.

There is no doubt that if I want to help someone, I need them to trust me. Very, very much.

It is not just a matter of transference neurosis, that artificial illness created in psychoanalysis to cure the original illness, as Sigmund Freud brilliantly put it in 1914. He noticed that patients developed very intense feelings towards him. Once he had quickly overcome the flattery of being a special person, he understood that it was a physiological and necessary event within a relationship as intimate as the analytical one. Far from considering it an accident or an obstacle, he made it the heart of the treatment. He encouraged its development. The analysis of transference neurosis could then resolve pathological neurotic conflicts. A lot has changed since then, but the fire continues to burn between patient and analyst, perhaps even more so.

A person can receive help in the attachment to their analyst. Very much so. But it is equally essential that the analyst loves the person sitting in front of them. Very much so.

Given these premises, the possible risk of crossing the line is high. Because on the one hand there is will and ethics, and on the other there are feelings, chemical and alchemical attractions, bodies and words that can make us feel so close.

The dangers of violating the setting lie on this impervious ridge.

But maybe we must first talk about seduction and its controversies.

Because the approach comes before the action.

Seduction has a dual nature: on the one hand, it leads to encounter, bonding, mutual attraction and desire, on the other, it is a source of danger surrounded by a harmful aura of mystery. Seduction, from the Latin *seducere*, composed of *se* ("apart, away") and *ducere* ("to lead, to draw"), means not only to attract, to charm, but also to lead away, off one's path, to distract, to distort, to incite evil with false reasons and deceit. Something harmful when applied to therapy.

In a certain sense, even the new psychoanalytic models, with their great attention to symmetrical relationships and reciprocity, can generate a shift in this direction.

But seduction is not limited to the realm of love and relationships: on the contrary, seduction has become hegemonic and widespread, infiltrating every area of social life. We live side by side with seduction.

We should not, therefore, demonise the society of seduction by idealising the past, but rather move towards a more creative development of seduction itself, limiting its pathogenic effects, sustaining its positive effects in the long term.

Gilles Lipovetsky, a French philosopher and sociologist, has been addressing these issues for some time. He argues that seduction can also be positive for people and society, creating an indispensable driving force that stimulates human action and the development of innovation and creativity. Thus, with less emphasis on appearance and illusion, often underlined in the past, seduction can be considered an indispensable component of the functioning of contemporary societies. Consequently, we should not fear or oppose seduction nor use it as a therapeutic tool, but rather, with conscious awareness we should try to understand and manage it. Every good psychotherapist knows that listening suddenly ceases when too much reality and too much action enter therapy. And when listening ceases there is no longer any cure or even any relationship. Whereas you can grant a space for seduction, even before it can be experienced, acted upon or suffered.

A more delicate point arises when it is not recognised. This can give rise to a new discord.

I remember the story of a young doctor, an aspiring psychiatrist at the time. He had been entrusted with teaching at the nursing school of a psychiatric hospital. On the sidelines of his classes, he had met a young psychologist who worked there. They met every week, chatted, and developed a mutual liking for each other. At the end of the day, the psychologist would reappear almost magically near the exit gate, driving her beloved and unmistakable Topolino, leaning out of the window and offering the doctor a lift to the railway station, which was not exactly nearby. The conversations resumed amiably until they said goodbye. This went on for weeks and months. Just words and rides. Many misunderstandings. Until the day when the psychologist decided to put a sign on the back of the car.

TAXI 5.

Actions speak louder than words.

I wonder if that young man, who later became a psychiatrist, finally learned how to recognise seduction.

One thing I am certain of, however. There is a big difference between reality and fantasy.

If a therapist knows this, he is safe.

And the red lights in his room will never come on.

12 Live or Die

As a recent graduate, I turned to a well-known training analyst. I wanted to start the training analysis as soon as possible to be able to become a psychoanalyst myself.

It was the first time I had been "on the other side of the desk", and it was a pleasant experience.

I remember some details very well, some words that touched me. I felt a sincere curiosity about my life, appreciation for my plan to pay for the therapy myself, attentive and respectful listening, but also sharp and incisive.

Here are some excerpts of the conversation.

"You are an intelligent person," he said as he took notes in a notebook.

Then he added: "But a bit of a *ruspin*…", a highly effective neologism, a mixture of dialects, Bergamasque and Milanese, to describe a way of being fussy, demanding, grumpy, difficult.

Finally, the conclusion: "You have just the right amount of pathology, neither too much nor too little, to undergo analysis and become a psychoanalyst." A verdict and a plan.

He advised me to begin personal analysis, postponing the didactic aspect until the appropriate time. Immediately called the colleague he considered most suitable and introduced me. A few days later, I saw my future therapist, who set the start of therapy for a year later. The deadline struck me. I don't know how psychoanalysts in the 1970s had such a precise idea of the end and beginning of analysis, sometimes even suggesting a five- or seven-year wait. They were different times.

During the interview, he also asked me if I had ever had suicidal thoughts. I was surprised but forced to look back on my teenage years and my moodiness from a new perspective.

Yes, death, depression, suicide. As this chapter took shape in my mind and on the keyboard, it began to seem to be an important memory and a necessary topic to address.

Psychoanalysis has long been considered a fad, suitable for bored ladies of high society, intellectuals or individuals who are already healthy. In reality, and without making too much fuss, we deal with people and their suffering, we deal with sensitive information, and this profession inevitably brings us

DOI: 10.4324/9781003759034-12

face to face with the risks of life and death. It constantly calls us to face our responsibilities. Responsibilities that cannot be delegated, but rest on our shoulders.

One story, among many, has always struck me as exemplary. The young heir of a wealthy Milanese family was ill. Due to a psychotic breakdown, he had fallen into an abyss of confusion, agitation, delirium and strangeness. He needed treatment, but as often happens with these conditions, he refused to accept.

The only hope now was hospitalisation. A willing young psychiatrist ventured into enemy territory, making a home visit in the hope of convincing the boy. His colleague had done well. The patient trusted him. With supportive parents and the clinic notified in advance, everything was ready for the journey of hope, the car was already on the road.

So, the small group got in, and guess how the crew arranged themselves?

The parents in the back seats, the psychiatrist in the passenger seat and the future patient, where else but behind the wheel? I know, it sounds like a joke, one of those "there was an Italian, a Frenchman and a German…" jokes. Unfortunately, it's true.

To be honest, this is the perfect example of how no one, none of those involved, had taken on responsibility.

Because proper respect for roles, skills and responsibilities would have required a different seating arrangement for the passengers. The patient and the psychiatrist in the back seats, with the lock-in device activated; the parents in the front seats, one of them driving.

It is true that doing this job also requires a certain amount of madness, recklessness and grandiosity, but defying the laws of common sense exceeds all permissible limits.

Can we predict or prevent suicide? Can we stop it?

As we know, a psychoanalyst is not a clairvoyant and does not possess crystal balls or divinatory abilities. The shiver that ran down my spine every time I sensed the proximity of a suicidal plan cannot be fully described or understood unless you have experienced it yourself. A moment that often coincides with our one and only chance to intervene.

It is not a question of becoming obsessed: living with fear makes us uncertain and fearful, which is the winning move in the ruthless strategy of terror that has been pursued since 2001 after the fall of the Twin Towers.

Our place lies between trust and caution. That is where we must learn to stand. Our minds must always be active, knowing that we may risk not identifying a suicidal plan in time, or underestimating that it represents the solution to their problems for many people. Think of how much adrenaline rushes through our veins when, for example during the summer, we leave our most delicate patients for our legitimate holidays. Nowadays, mobile phones and emails keep us potentially always connected and within reach, but how did psychoanalysts manage with their at-risk patients in the past? Perhaps now we delude ourselves into thinking that we can always control what happens around us. This is not the case.

I have always been convinced that no one can prevent a person from committing suicide. Someone compares it to having the right to freely choose when to end one's life. Taking this consideration into account can be realistic and healthy, even protective of ourselves. Because unfortunately it happens, however it happens.

And then there is the aftermath to deal with.

I fear I do not have the words to describe it, beyond the dismay, the guilt, the fear of having done the wrong thing, the emptiness that follows. I never cross out the appointments in the diary reserved for patients who die, regardless of if caused by suicide or not. They remain there for a long time as if they were sacred. A form of respect, a tribute. The same as in sports, when a player's number who was the symbol of a team has retired.

Finally, time eases the pain. At least a little.

We are powerless, as I said before, but it does not mean we should not try anyway.

With intuition, even the most unconscious.

Francesca was 16 years old. Shortly before, she had lost her mother to illness. Despite having a father who loved her, she could no longer find any reason to live. She drifted through empty days, dropping out of school, with few relationships. And she was determined to die. Her suicide plans and attempts had necessitated a first hospitalisation, then a second. Therapeutic failures and protective interventions followed one after another. The minimum goal was to at least make it difficult for her to harm herself. It was an endless escalation with limited purpose.

She had been sent to me for therapy. She was still hospitalised, always accompanied by a "guardian". In the sessions, her script repeated itself incessantly without change. "There's no point in living, I want to die, leave me to my fate, I can't take it anymore!" My interventions no longer varied, nor were they effective. We couldn't talk about anything else. I was completely powerless.

One particularly dark day for me, after yet another repetition of the familiar litany, exasperated but convinced, I said to her: "All right, Francesca, I understand what you're saying, and I realise you can't take it anymore. But I still see it differently. So, I propose a deal: if you convince me that this is really the right solution, the best one for you, I'll help you die. In the meantime, though, let's try to work together a little. Are you in?" She agreed, and we finally began therapy, which continued for a few years. We never spoke of our agreement again.

One day, as the end of the treatment was approaching and Francesca had resumed her life, school, relationships and even her affections, she stopped and asked me, "Doctor, can I ask you a question? When you made that proposal to me years ago, that agreement… but… but… were you serious?"

Marta – Thursday, 4.45 p.m.

On 20 August, I climbed up to the eighth floor because I wanted to throw myself down.

I stood on the railing, with one leg outside and one inside, perfectly balanced. I don't know for how long.

I was in a trance. The city didn't even look like Milan from up there. Fog.

I had put a note in a plastic folder so that it wouldn't get stained with my blood during the impact. Call Fabio Bianchi, I had written. My most trusted friend. I had added a number. And a message: *I'm finally happy again.* I had also put my house keys inside.

Everything was ready.

I tied the plastic folder to my wrist with a cord I had bought in India the previous winter. All I had to do was step over the railing with my other leg and I would fall. It could have been over in an instant, but I couldn't do it. As much as I wanted to, despite the certainty that it was the best solution for everyone, for me, since I would never recover and would suffer unbearably forever, and for my family, who would have to take care of me for the rest of their lives.

So, it was right, right in my head, but I couldn't do it.

Damn survival instinct. At that moment, it was holding me back. But I knew how to trick it.

I went home. I took ten drops of the anti-anxiety drug En. I smoked my last cigarette.

When I felt the medicine taking effect, I got up, walked towards the door, still with my plastic folder on my wrist, and just as I was about to open it, my mobile rang.

I remember answering it. I remember it was my psychiatrist.

I don't remember what I said to him, vaguely what he said to me.

"In the state you're in, go straight to the emergency room of the nearest hospital. Do you think you can do it?"

Without thinking, I obeyed. I was still in a trance. I looked like a robot carrying out an order.

I remember taking some €50 banknotes I had at home and putting them in my pocket.

I remember walking to the tobacconist's, buying packets of cigarettes, I don't even know how many, to change the money, and then getting into a taxi.

I remember telling the driver to take me to the emergency room. Nothing else.

I don't remember sending Fabio a message telling him I was going to the hospital because I was about to do something stupid. But I did.

I got out of the taxi, smoked a cigarette, and waited for my friend to arrive. I was shaking. I didn't realise anything.

When I finished the cigarette, I heard the doctor's words again.

"In the state you're in, go straight to the emergency room." So, I rushed in. There was no one else in line. I got to the counter, said something, I don't know what, and a second later I found myself in front of a nurse who was trying to reassure me. He said I would be better very soon. That the doctor was coming. He also brought me a glass of water and sugar. I didn't speak. I either nodded or shook my head, depending on what I was asked. And I kept shaking. Then I found myself in a room talking to a doctor with short blonde hair. She explained that the beds in the hospital were all full and that they would transfer me. I also vaguely remember a lot of doctors watching me and asking me questions.

I couldn't say what. I answered, but I don't know what. I don't remember anything else until I entered the ward.

From then on, I only retained fragments, blurred, unreal images in my memory, like a terrible nightmare. There was a man wandering around in striped pyjamas. He had a trail of drool etched on his face at least 15 centimetres long, perfectly still as he paced back and forth down the corridor. Another was screaming and banging his head and his hands on the wall, with all the rage he could muster up, and he didn't seem to want to stop. A lady came up to me. She was bent over, but she had no physical deformities. She was crippled with pain. She was writhing with absurd movements and wanted some of the fruit salad I was eating, I don't know why. And without knowing why, I fed her with my spoon.

In the middle of the night, I heard noises and hellish screams.

My neighbour in my bedroom had been tied up and was being taken away from the room.

The man in the corridor kept banging on the wall and hitting himself.

The deformed woman was banging on the walls because she couldn't walk straight.

While I stood paralysed at my bedroom door, another woman came out: she stood in the middle of the corridor, and she sang "Jesus will protect us" in an angelic voice that at that moment seemed to have been sent by the devil himself.

I don't remember how, but I went back to sleep.

The second time I woke up, I had a needle in my vein. First, I saw the needle, and then the nurse. It was just for blood tests, and I had to stay calm and still.

"Yes, good, that's it. Done." I was still in a trance.

A few hours earlier, I had been truly happy, feeling finally liberated, light and relieved at the mere thought of dying. I already felt dead.

Even before I thought about suicide, part of me was truly dead forever. To make way for my dark side. We all have one. I was literally possessed by it. I called it *Dolores*.

That pain that tears your soul into a thousand pieces as if it were wastepaper. I said that *Dolores* had returned and possessed me. For the first time, in the hospital, I became aware of it. In those last few months, I had lost my identity without even knowing how or why. An infinite and profound world lay before me, incredibly structured, that I had never seen before.

Dolores' face is the opposite of mine.

I smile; I have very white teeth and dark skin. People often mistake me for an Indian.

She is gloomy, pale, with yellowish, neglected teeth. She is depression.

That's how we are. Not everyone, but at least that's how I am. And now I know. I know a lot of things I didn't know before.

I know that to be reborn, you must die.

I know that dying hurts a lot. I know that you can be aware of being dead while you are alive.

I know that you can go into a trance without taking drugs. I know that you can be truly happy to die.

I know that there is an infinite world inside me, and I know that my dark side now needs all my attention to become clearer and clearer.

I know that mad people are mad because they have a dysfunction. I know that mood control is a function of certain neurotransmitters that make you feel normal, and when they go haywire, you go haywire. Your short-term memory goes haywire, completely, to make room for long-term memory, the one that makes you remember when you were little, little. Your sense of pleasure, serenity, calmness goes to hell, and everything becomes extremely difficult. It's like having a lot of people in your head. You hear voices. They are your thoughts, but there are too many of them and they go too fast to keep up with. You hear your brain throbbing like the heart of a marathon runner at the end of a race. You can feel it burning. You feel that you can no longer distinguish between right and wrong, and then you feel that everything negative is reality, and the world you had been living in until two seconds ago, the one you liked, is just an illusion. You know that your perception has gone to hell, and so you are totally thrown off balance by everything, even the most insignificant things. You know you are at the mercy of a self you have never known before. And you feel bad. So bad that it is unbearable. With no way out. Because every evil can be fought rationally, but without your brain you are defenceless. You are barehanded in front of a fire that is engulfing you.

And you can't wait for it to be over. There it is madness. Naked and raw, in all its forms. This was mine. I didn't know how, but I had gone mad.

Can a love that has ended reduce you in these conditions? It happened to me.

I curled up and cried in "that" way: the way that mad people do when they know they are already dead and have no way out except to destroy the container, that is, the bloody body that, in the end, becomes a sadistic executioner that keeps them under torture.

The sadistic container ended up in the psychiatric ward of a hospital.

The next morning, I received a text message from my psychotherapist. It was gently paternal: "Trust and rely on their care," he wrote. I trusted him;

he was the only one who could understand what was happening to me a thousand times better than I could. And, as always, I obeyed.

Once a day, Dr R. would come to the ward. He was very kind and, fortunately, very good at his job. He was also young, but he understood me immediately, and I understood him right away. I understood him because he could read my mind and anticipate what I was going to say before I even knew it myself. Sometimes he even scared me. Dr R. listened first. Then he gave advice but always leaving me free to do things my way. I had to let go of everything that had caused me to break down. I had to accept my weakness. I had to accept my illness. I had to accept that I was not who I thought I was.

So, I started again from scratch. One thing at a time, taking my time.

Dr R. told me what my psychotherapist had already told me, and what I already knew myself. I was unable to ask for help and, even when I did, it was too late, when I had already hurt myself. So, I had to learn to ask for help in time.

That morning, I hadn't done so.

I had to learn to protect and defend myself. I had never managed to do so.

I shouldn't be ashamed of doing so, nor should I feel guilty. That was the real key. I was ashamed and felt guilty because I didn't think I deserved all that love, all that attention.

"Go out, get your life back, go out there," Dr R. told me one morning.

"But do you know how hard it is to be different from everyone else, every day, all day long? I'm different, I know that now, I'm like the people in this ward, and I want to stay here. I can't go back out there, I'm already in too much pain, I can't take it anymore."

I stopped nervously curling my sock and leaned back against the headboard.

Dr R. smiled at me. He was always calm.

"Your place is out there, and you know it. Right now, you can't do it, but that's exactly why you must go out. The more you get used to being here, the harder it will be to leave. If you break down, we'll pull you out. But now you must go back out there. Your brother is coming tomorrow. Go out with him, go home, and come back here in the afternoon. If something goes wrong, if you panic or if you don't feel up to it, come here first, OK?"

I just nodded. I knew he was right.

It was strange. I opened the door, and my home looked beautiful to me. Much more beautiful than I remembered it. It may seem strange, but before I went to the eighth floor to throw myself off, I had cleaned and tidied everything up so maniacally, getting rid of a lot of old and useless things. I needed to see that everything could be put back in its place, and since I couldn't do it inside myself, I started doing it outside. It made me feel better. And now, seeing my house so beautifully colourful, tidy and clean, I felt a sense of calm.

Back in the ward, Dr R. had an even calmer smile than usual.

"OK, tomorrow I'll let you out again, but not completely. Let's call it conditional freedom. OK?"

"OK."

"Please, ask for help. Before you hurt yourself, not after. And don't be a cyborg. You're very good. Really. You're really, really good."

"Really?"

"Of course."

"Thank you, Doctor, thank you, from the bottom of my heart. I really want to get better."

"I know. You're already healing and you've made great strides. It's been a real pleasure working with you."

The next day, I was in my psychiatrist's office. My parole allowed me to resume sessions with him. The last time we spoke, he saved my life. And now I was there.

When I called him on 20 August, he was cycling. He couldn't answer his mobile phone. He stopped a few kilometres later, in a clearing, to check his calls and saw that it was me.

I had never called him before; I was always afraid of disturbing him.

But this time I had made that choice.

He called me back just as the drops of En had taken effect and I was about to go back to the eighth floor. Just in time to tell me to rush to the emergency room. Right away. Immediately. A phone call saves your life. Two seconds later, it would have been too late.

I am certain that I would have killed myself. I am so sure for one simple reason. If I had done it just to free myself, it's true, I wouldn't have succeeded, because I didn't love myself enough. But I was driven by the desire to free all the people I loved from me.

Thanks to those two seconds, I am still here. Pulling the thread of my skein. And now that I have it before my eyes, my enemy, I know it well. By now, I understand how it works, but I still have a long way to go. I must stop feeling wrong. I must stop taking on responsibilities that aren't mine and stop always wanting to be strong, stronger than others, and wanting to protect them all the time and at all costs. And then I must learn to ask for help.

To let myself be pampered. To let myself be protected. To listen to myself so I don't hurt myself anymore. To let myself go. Above all, I must learn to love myself. To do myself good.

I have to rebuild everything from the ground up. I will do it.

It will take a lot of time and a lot of effort, but I want to do it. I want to heal. I want to fall asleep again at night with a smile in my eyes and wake up like that the next day. I want my lightness back. I want to be happy and make those around me happy. I want everything I never thought I deserved.

The Analyst and Antonella – Thursday and Monday, 5.45 p.m.

I wonder if that boy leaning out of the window still remembers the scene.

What happens to certain frightening, irreversible images that are imprinted on our retinas like ink etchings?

Forgetting seems like a good strategy. If you can do it. I still can't do it today, many years later, even though I wasn't there.

There is one thing I have learned for sure, and I don't know if it's enough: to be very careful, even more careful than usual, with people who ask for an appointment as the holidays approach.

It may be a coincidence, of course, but it is still something to keep in mind. Always.

I haven't taken off my work clothes yet. So, when Antonella contacts me for an appointment, I feel ready and curious to meet her.

Finding a day and time is not easy. It's not that I'm playing hard to get, it's that she can't get away from her professional commitments. In the end, with a few mutual compromises, we manage to set a date.

Something about Antonella struck me from the very first contact. I still don't know what it was, or what it will be, that makes her so special to me. Perhaps the fact that she was sent by a friend of hers whom I had helped with a parenting problem and whom I remember fondly. When I meet her, I get a positive feeling: she is direct, physically healthy, I would describe her as a simple beauty.

"Eva spoke very highly of you, she said you can help me, that I should take this as a nice gift to myself."

It took a lot to make this decision. If it were up to her, she would always try to make it on her own.

It is an excellent meeting, warm and affectionate, despite the initial difficulties.

Antonella has done everything she could in life. At least so far.

Her family is originally from Eastern Europe, she tells me, but she was born in Milan, where her parents moved many years ago. It was her father, a very ambitious man, who chose Milan to develop his business activities. She tells me about her younger brother, eight years less than her, her loving mother with whom she is very close, and her turbulent adolescence. Panic attacks began when she started university: she was referred to a psychiatrist, whom she met about ten times. Despite the difficulties, she talks about a brilliant academic career, interspersed with a period abroad, a master's degree in another city, and finally a job at a large company in Milan, exactly where she hoped to end up. It is the typical educational path of many talented and determined young women today. As I listen to her, I compare her story with that of my daughter, who is the same age.

Antonella's romantic relationships, on the other hand, appear much more complicated. Three very important relationships: the first with a boy her own age, in which she submitted herself to violent dynamics; the second, during her time abroad, marked by the fantasy/risk of pregnancy, with a man that was younger than her, whom she describes as her great love; the last, during her master's degree, with a psychologically unstable partner. All these relationships ended badly.

I feel her loneliness, almost lost. And as I listen to her first stories, a multitude of feelings stir within me.

Like in the opening moves of a chess game, I must choose which pieces to use in my strategy, where to focus my attention. I choose the theme of "pregnancy". It is not clear to me what happened, what fantasies were triggered, how it ended and why it was so traumatic. We talk about it at length. She is happy to do so.

Antonella remembers that her period was late, which was unusual for her as she was always so regular in her physiological cycles, as in life. At first, she thought it was due to her recent move, and she wasn't particularly worried, but after a month she decided to do a pregnancy test. The positive result came as a shock. However, Antonella was able to count on her mother for her understanding and support, while she decided that the man she was dating was too young to share this event. She felt lost, totally unable to decide. Keeping the baby was the option closest to her moral convictions, but terminating the pregnancy seemed to be the most logical choice on a rational level. The impossibility of making a choice distressed her terribly.

Fate, or whatever you want to call it, had decided for her: going to the bathroom one morning, she had seen, with terror and relief at the same time, the beginnings of a life that was starting inside her body disappear into the toilet, in that clot of blood.

Antonella had experienced that miscarriage – clinically it was an ectopic pregnancy – as a voluntary act, a choice for which she took full responsibility. And although she was aware that what had happened simplified her life, she felt she was returning to a period of dependence and regression: "When I had the operation, all the other women had their boyfriend or husband or a friend with them, but I had my mother with me."

She decided to seek help, she explains, because shortly after starting her new job, which coincided with her return to Milan and her family, she felt ill, her panic attacks returned, she suffered from insomnia, and she feared she would not be able to cope.

When Antonella goes on to tell me about her job, about the difficulties in her relationship with a boss who not only fails to recognise her abilities and skills but even seems to want to undermine and attack her, I sense a shift in her, she seems to become despondent and it cannot be explained solely by a conflict, albeit an unpleasant one, with her superior.

Immediately afterwards, she confesses that because of these difficulties, she often fantasises about escaping, imagining assignments in foreign countries, even working on humanitarian projects. But she herself recognises the escapist nature of these fantasies. She is certainly a very intelligent and determined young woman, I think to myself, when she tells me that another fantasy has accompanied her since adolescence: that of suicide. However, she reassures me that these thoughts have never taken the form of an actual plan.

At the end of the interview, I tell her that I have some good news and some bad news. The good news is that there is a real possibility of helping her with the various tools we have at our disposal (however, Antonella is very wary of the possibility of resorting to medication); the bad news is related to the upcoming holidays. She does not seem surprised. I offer her the chance to meet again in a week, before my departure, but she can't make it, so we find a slot four days later and set the appointment.

As she leaves, she does not ask me for my fee. A few minutes later, she calls me to apologise for her oversight. No big deal: we will see each other again soon, and I am sure she will not run away.

She arrives on time for the second meeting, looking much more polished and elegant. She tells me she is feeling better and has finally slept.

She immediately mentions our phone call and her failure to pay.

"I wonder what you thought of me, careless and annoying."

"Do you really want to know what I thought?"

"Of course!"

"I thought that perhaps you had been quite struck by our meeting – which could explain your forgetfulness. You were, after all, a conscientious and respectful person – which is why you had notified me immediately – and perhaps you wanted to see if I would answer your phone call."

She smiles, as if to say she agrees.

"Over the last two days, I've thought a lot about my family relationships. I really didn't think they were still so important to me. Maybe I still can't do without them…"

Then, suddenly, she starts talking about work again.

"I've had more conflicts. I felt very humiliated when, after offering my complete availability to finish a job, my boss told me I was presumptuous and arrogant because it was up to them to decide if, how and when they needed me."

I imagined what it must be like to work in a hostile environment, where you are not recognised, and the frustration and pain that this causes.

We talked about it for a while.

"You know what? You're just like the man in the film *Caos calmo*. You sit there on the bench, watching people go by and waiting for those who need you."

I look at her in surprise. Questioningly.

"I read your comment on the film on the SPI website. I liked it."

I'm taken aback, I don't know how to react, I feel confused.

"It's a reassuring image, but perhaps a little passive, don't you think?"

Antonella drops the subject. And the interview is about to end. It has been intense, engaging, challenging. I feel that many doors have opened, perhaps too many, and I also think about how many things will remain pending. I try to suggest another appointment during the week, the last one before the summer holidays.

"I can't, I have too much work, too many things to finish and sort out."

She asks me for an appointment in September anyway. I'm not at ease.

This happens to me when our meetings in the room seem to be both "easy" and "suspended" at the same time. Why did she ask for an appointment right now? If she has made up her mind, why is she finding it so difficult to find a flicker of possibility? Our meeting, she said, seems to have opened important thoughts and reflections for her. So why doesn't she want to continue, even for a short time, but postpone everything until after the summer? Intuitively, I sense a hidden or concealed desire to escape. Perhaps it would be the same at another time of year, but at this moment it seems almost threatening. How can I tell her? "Will I see you again in September?" I ask her sadly. Antonella doesn't answer me.

"So let me explain how I organise myself during holiday periods, how and when you can contact me by telephone or email."

"Thank you, but I don't want to take advantage of you. I'm afraid of becoming dependent, I don't like being dependent."

"I imagine this is a sensitive issue for you; we also talked about it in relation to your mother and your family. But it's also true that if we don't accept our needs, it's difficult to become stronger, don't you think?"

She smiles at me.

Our time is up. She asks me about the fee. She doesn't have any cheques, and I don't have a card machine. I'll send her the invoice by email.

We say goodbye.

The following Monday, after a quiet weekend, Antonella leaves the house early in the morning.

She must go to work. She has important meetings. She takes her bag and leaves her mobile phone on the bedside table.

Instead of going down the stairs of the building, she goes up to the top floor. Very high up.

She opens the ventilation window overlooking the inner courtyard.

She sits on the frame.

Nothing separates her from the void. No ledge, no railing.

She hesitates for a moment.

She catches the eye of a boy leaning out of the window of the building on the opposite side.

Then she lets herself fall. Without a cry.

Without a farewell note. Without a reason.

Post

I heard from Eva, the friend who had sent her, and offered to meet Antonella's relatives. Farewell ceremonies, like funerals, are helpful for the living, for those who survive. That was the case here, for me and for them. The meeting, a heartfelt and poignant conversation with her parents, took place on Ferragosto. We had never met before. It was a unique and unrepeatable occasion.

We found ourselves sharing our dismay, pain and loss. Without resentment, without anger.

Words and feelings came, unprepared by anyone, necessary for everyone.

Many memories, many questions that did not require answers. Just sharing and respect.

It was one of the most painful and intense conversations that room has ever hosted.

And one of the most useful. For everyone.

The Analyst and Class 2° C of a Milanese High School – Friday, 8.00 a.m.[1]

When I entered that classroom, a yellow room with white neon lighting and a grey sky outside, there was a red rose on the green desk. Scarlet. Like the blood now clotted on the pavement, because what we all had before our eyes was the *Corriere*, a large photo on page 15 of the Italian news, a dark stain on the asphalt. From the bottom corner, the ATM transportation card of a 16-year-old who had fallen from the fourteenth floor still stared at us, without a message, without a reason.

Can we really believe what we don't understand? What can't we explain?

Two days earlier, there had already been a suicide in another city. Just trying to say that maybe something was happening. Or maybe not. I agreed without hesitation when a colleague asked me to speak to the class of the boy who had died – it's one of our practices, it's called *postvention*. I'm a psychiatrist. I'm an expert. I know what to do, I know what to expect. I know where I want to go.

It was a grey, rainy day, with that pale light that seems to weigh on the city, clouding the streets, blurring the outlines of buildings, rendering reality two-dimensional: flattened against a washed-out backdrop, not even the sounds of the tram can pierce the surface. I even wondered if I had gone deaf. It was as if we had all gone deaf.

I enter the classroom cautiously, 20 or more waxy faces staring at me. I am used to observing carefully, so I see sweatshirts and jumpers, exaggerated make-up and piercings, tattered backpacks and tidy totes, I see necklaces, strands of hair covering eyes and glasses hiding pain. Then the red rose, and I stop in front of the desk. I get the idea to start from there.

I introduce myself, briefly explain what we will be doing in the programmed hour and a half, and proceed cautiously, asking simple questions. There is a kind of door between today and tomorrow, I try to say. Today we are prisoners of dismaying thoughts. Beyond that door lies what we will become. Perhaps something better.

Let's try to get there together. I try to listen to them one by one. At each desk, I slow down, as if I were facing a bend in a river or an uphill climb. Suddenly, someone throws the one big question right at me, the one that can crush me.

"Don't you think we've already asked ourselves these questions? We were here, where the hell were you, what do you know?"

Wow, I didn't expect that so soon. I am quite familiar with this question; it always comes up. It hurts as much as ever.

Slowly, step by step, I weave my way through the escape routes of their anger. I try not to rush. Perhaps my emotion is also visible. Then someone gives in. And the tears come. Someone else gets up and leaves. After a while, they come back. Another even manages to make a joke.

In the end, I encounter tougher resistance: a blonde girl with wild dreadlocks, two eye-catching bracelets that never stopped rattling in the classroom, a bluish vein on her forehead, bright eyes and a broken voice. She is his friend, his friend. Until now, she has been silent and aloof. Distrustful. Now she openly attacks me, everyone.

She stands up and confronts me with a piece of paper in her hands. He wrote it. A few days ago. Neat, delicate handwriting, a scrap from a notebook.

I read it: a thought that illuminates the scene.

"Some nights I lie awake dreaming of a better life, which does not exist. It is even easier to close my eyes forever and never dream."

In hindsight, it seems like the formulation of a plan, a kind of message in a bottle, not thrown into the sea but entrusted to a sailor. Where has it been until now? Where did his friend keep it? How many times did she read and reread it? How did she feel each time? Guilt, as we know, destroys everyone.

I don't know how we dealt with it all, or maybe I do, but I don't remember it well. It seemed like improvisation, but I was fully aware of what was happening, thanks to a mixture of experience and common sense, which always helps. You always come out of these storms shipwrecked, with no idea where you'll end up, but at least we got there together. It was precisely by being together that we made it, I think. It was at that precise moment that I was able to get close to them, with them, among them. No longer an "expert" who knew everything, but an adult who came down from the lectern, sat among the desks, really, and tried to understand what seemed incomprehensible and unspeakable. To everyone. We said goodbye with the sun cutting the air in half, illuminating the incessant dust dance in the crowded classroom, the chairs scraping on the floor: some left their desks to say goodbye to me, others reopened their books, others continued their morning as if nothing had happened.

When I went outside, the sky had cleared, the sun was shining, and at the tram stop I wasn't thinking about anything anymore. It was as if I had no thoughts left. And no light either. It was as if all the shadows from that classroom had stuck onto my jacket.

Taking my clothes off wouldn't be enough to get rid of them. That was the only thought I remember having.

Then darkness again. And an experience I will never forget.

Note

1 Written with Armando Barone, "Omeostasi", blog from "La settimana corta", 9/1/2015, subject to personal reworking.

13 What Will Become of Them… and of Me?

The Analyst and Sara – Friday, 9.45 a.m.

A few hours have passed since our first meeting.

I'm still working, but the feelings Sara left in me reverberate like beams of light in the dark. Sudden, immediate, pleasant and painful at the same time.

During a break, I open my Mac, and an icon flashes in the upper right corner. Mail.

I click, I see, another click. I open it. I read it.

I would simply like to thank you. Because our meeting this morning represented a turning point for me: a point of arrival, a point of departure, a turning point, I don't know. I only know that it has a very strong, almost overwhelming significance. And I think that's wonderful, even if it's within a professional relationship, knowing that you were important at a key moment in another person's life. Thank you.

Sara's email fills the screen, together with her words and the emotions they stir in me.

The words are a new flash of light. A confirmation of harmony. Perhaps too much harmony.

I think back on our meeting in my memory. The memories are close at hand.

A young woman who, with modestly but with great determination, asks for help in dealing with her current difficulties. It is not easy to imagine her struggling with problems. She is pleasant, intelligent, friendly, introspective, helpful. Her academic record would arouse the interest of any headhunter. A degree in philosophy with top grades, a master's degree abroad at a prestigious university. Her return to Italy, getting a job that was exactly what she dreamed of. A satisfying social, emotional and romantic life.

So, what brought her to a psychoanalyst's office? I still don't know. Sara must be one of those people who gracefully guard their discomfort: she doesn't hide it out of a need to appear different, perhaps better than what she really is. There is no duplicity in her. Rather, it is a habit of stepping aside, a desire not to cause concern or pity in others. But you can see the pain in her eyes, black and deep, but slightly downturned, with a melancholic

DOI: 10.4324/9781003759034-13

expression; in her slightly forward-leaning posture, strange and suspicious in a woman with a slender physique; on a gym mat, "I have to stretch every day, otherwise my back won't hold up…" And then, being so pretty, why doesn't she make the most of her appearance with her clothing?

The discomfort she mentions seems to have appeared shortly after she achieved her objectives, as if she wasn't allowed to enjoy her finally hard-won victories, the fruit of several sacrifices. What had happened in her past and inside herself to prevent her from doing so? I ask her the question delicately. I get no answers, only attention. That's something.

For a while during our first conversation, it almost felt like I was talking to an acquaintance, a travelling companion, as on the train or airport waiting rooms.

Then, suddenly, the scenario changed bringing us into a new dimension.

The conversation we were having was interrupted, a prolonged silence fell between us, her gaze lost in the void.

"What's going on, Sara?" Another brief hesitation.

"There's something I've never told anyone, something I've carried inside myself for almost my entire life… I never thought I'd be able to talk about it… but now it's coming out, like an unstoppable need…"

"I'm glad you feel you can do it here and now. I'm with you. I'm ready."

Thus, she begins the long story of abuse perpetrated by a relative, which began when she was just a child and continued for many years, until she reached adolescence. Sara seems like a river that's flooding, but calm and proud in its flow. Although it could have seemed like a flood, I had a sense of relief as if a giant plug was finally being removed freeing the turbulent waters held back by a dam.

Sometimes, almost unimaginable conditions arise in our studies.

As the emotional impact of the stories we hear increases, we feel as if immersed in high-temperature thermal pools fed by geysers. There are some moments when it is impossible to remain impervious when the stories we hear affect us so deeply.

Towards the end of the interview, the emotional flow has calmed down a little. We have managed to bring the temperature of the environment back to acceptable levels. The story has slowly become less vehement, less painful. The water basin has almost emptied, no longer exhorting pressure on her, leaving room for more structured thinking.

We made a second appointment. In conclusion, I suggested starting of a course of therapy. Calmly. Sara agreed.

She was happy. She seemed happy.

The following week, the day before our scheduled meeting, I received a text message from her.

"Unfortunately, I must cancel the appointment due to a work commitment outside the city. I'll get in touch as soon as I get back."

I had no reason to suspect lies or excuses. Cancellations or rescheduling of sessions are now commonplace. Our schedules are unstable. We seem to be getting used to it; these are no longer the times of absolute loyalty and stability, when patients did not feel entitled to ask to reschedule a session and any missed sessions were still charged at the end of the month. There are urban legends about a patient who had to pay for her sessions during the period, when she had been kidnapped in the 1970s. Excesses, abuses. Definitely.

With Sara, in this case, as I always do, I wondered if there could be other reasons besides work. I left the question unanswered.

My doubts became certainties in the weeks that followed. This time, it was an email.

Doctor, I want to tell you that I am fine. Thank you again for our meeting, for what it meant to me. As for the therapy, I don't feel ready to start it yet. I would like to think about it some more. I want to see how things go.

Several years ago, at the beginning of my career, when another patient sent me a similar letter (there were no text messages or emails back then), I wrote in my notebook: "She'll be back." I never saw her again.

This time, however, I was certain that I would never see Sara again. An easy prediction by now.

All right. I understand and respect your decision, even though I'm sorry, because I would have enjoyed working with you. Please know that I'm still here.

A mistake, then? A failure? Where did I go wrong? What could I have done differently?

Unanswered questions, but necessary ones.

What if that first and only meeting was enough for Sara?

A turning point: a point of arrival, a point of departure, a turning point, I don't know.

There are occasions when the parameters of psychoanalysis are questioned or even overturned. More sessions each week? Years of treatment? Unaffordable costs?

Not always.

Sara had certainly managed to ask, to tell her story; she had been listened to, she had felt understood, seen and, I believe, recognised. Ultimately, this is what we need to feel better, even if I don't feel comfortable saying that a single session is enough. Perhaps, and I repeat, perhaps, for her, at that moment in her life, it represented something important, something new, something that finally allowed her to feel at peace with such a painful past.

I do not know where Sara is or who she is now. What had become of her, if indeed, as Owen Renik amiably recounts, psychoanalysis is possible in a single session. What had our exchange left inside her, what results had it produced.

***

One of the concerns of every analyst is the fate of the people they have accompanied for a part of their lives. Where are they? How are they? What has become of them? Are they married? Separated? Had children? Grown up? How? Did that dream or that project come true? What will become of that aspiring actress? And the journalist, the teacher, the student? Or the dreamer?

Yes, what happens to the people we talk to after we meet them?

Not knowing how their stories end is the most frequent among the many frustrations of my job. When a person leaves my room for the last time, whether after one, two or a thousand sessions, it's all over. Their life, the one they will live from then on, will remain a mystery to me. As if we were two strangers. Which we are not.

Everyone of them, more or less explicitly, ask me to help them to rewrite their story. And I know from experience, that to be able to do so, you must reach a very high level of intimacy, sometimes even comparable to that of an emotional, almost loving bond. When a person leaves my professional life forever, it is as if a child, respectfully and lovingly accompanied as they grow up, were leaving home. Pride and sorrow at the same time.

I often fantasised about sending letters to old patients. Something to do perhaps in old age, when the past and its memories become more fleeting and at the same time more important. I then discovered that it was not such an original fantasy, especially when I came across Robert U. Akeret (*The Man Who Fell in Love with a White Bear*), an American psychoanalyst who, at the age of 66 (younger than me at the moment…), after more than 40 years of analytical practice, decided to take a break from his work to visit some of his patients, whom he had discharged several years earlier, to find out where they were and what the analysis had brought to their lives. Perhaps also to understand if he had "really" been helpful. He gets into a Plymouth Voyager and sets off on an extraordinary journey (the original title was "Tales from a Travelling Couch") searching for the end of the stories. He recounts five of them, fascinating and not necessarily exemplary. Then he returns to his work, with even more doubts than when he left, but with an answer about the effectiveness of psychoanalysis provided by a former patient.

"Maybe it works only when it works." And that's enough for him.

With this statement, I do not wish to belittle the indispensable and complex research on the effectiveness of analysis, especially the questions about "What works (and doesn't) for whom, how and when?" Nor do I wish to belittle the factors that make it therapeutic. On the contrary, they are welcome and should be communicated. They are useful to everyone, patients and analysts alike.

I think, again and again, of that sense of frustration and uncertainty at the end of therapy.

Perhaps we are just ferrymen who transport travellers along the stretch of road or for the time they need, picking them up from one shore, with more or less ease, and taking them to their destination, wherever they want to go. And then we return, like shuttles, to the starting point, ready for another journey. A valuable and reassuring function, if we think of the panic attacks experienced by some passengers when they realise they are travelling on automatic shuttles without a pilot or driver. In some cases, they experience such intense and unmanageable crises that it has become necessary to have staff on board to reassure lost and uncertain travellers. It is better to be accompanied.

Perhaps I am just an incurable romantic who cannot bear to be equated with a function. Perhaps I find it difficult to accept the possibility of being, I won't say forgotten but having a less decisive role and priority in a person's life.

In any case, this is a condition that must be accepted, notwithstanding exceptional pathetic scenes or clandestine operations. I know of colleagues who scour the web or social networks in search of news about former patients, their stories, and the outcomes of distant therapies. As can be seen, this is not so different from more or less successful attempts to find information on the internet about old youthful loves. Often producing risky consequences.

I confess that I too sometimes find myself rummaging through WhatsApp profile pictures, curious to see what the people I have met over the years look like now and, I won't deny it, to catch a glimpse of their lives.

It is undeniable that we are all children of our time. In any case, in these cases, the encounter is only virtual. Whereas meeting face to face, patient and analyst, is a real and potentially extremely intimate experience.

This happened to me not long ago. My wife and I were invited to an informal dinner by a dear mutual friend, and we were happy and curious about the company we would find. Arriving slightly late, we noticed that two extra places had been set at the table. Time passed, the food was almost ready, but the absent guests did not show up. With some embarrassment, our hostess finally informed us that the two missing guests, who had arrived before us, had left once they learned that "the Goisis'" would be among the guests – "And he's the psychoanalyst?", "Yes, why?" – and that they had left the house in a hurry.

A funny anecdote, perhaps. But also, a little frustrating. Mysterious, too.

Most of the time, I must settle for the traces that people have left behind in the room. In addition to objects, thoughts, memories and recollections, there are the many signs that I have constructed and created.

Mainly writings, diagrams, notes. Handwritten sheets and files on my Mac.

I know that our notes are one of the myths, and one of the problems, of our work.

The analysts and the notes they take have such a personal quality that it is almost difficult to talk about it. Sometimes with maniacal and obsessive care, especially at the beginning of the work, dedicating as much time to them as to the sessions themselves. Especially if they are intended for meetings with supervisors. Sometimes with irritation, a necessary obligation. Carving out space from life and sleep. It is best to write them down immediately, while the memory is still fresh. Never during interviews, if possible. Or else they can be made up of fragments, coded phrases, hieroglyphics to be deciphered if they end up in the hands of others. A sort of extremely personal conceptual map that is useful only to us. Some use computers, some use loose sheets of paper, some use notebooks that accumulate in bookcases year after year.

On the one hand, they contain our thoughts about the people we meet often with genuine descriptions, without filters. Sometimes they refer to what stimulates us, our instinctive reactions, our striking comments. Even if we don't write them down, they often remain etched in our minds almost surprising the patients themselves, who more than once ask us, "You don't take notes… how do you remember everything I tell you?" Then there are the pages that are more structured, consisting of entire transcribed sessions, actual clinical reports, reports of verbal and non-verbal exchanges. These are valuable objects of study, intended for refined research and complex reflections on the meaning of our profession and its effectiveness. I imagine you might want to have a little taste of them. It's best to know in advance that it won't be like reading a detective or adventure novel. Here is an excerpt from the transcript of a session from many years ago. Today I would use different words and methods, but this is what happened back then.

Monday, 28 May.

She arrives five minutes late. She is out of breath, apologises, enters the room and quickly sits down in her armchair. She seems lost in thought. She looks straight ahead, avoiding my gaze.

Ten minutes of silence.

"I won't be very talkative today because I've been to the dentist, he gave me an anaesthetic and devitalised a nerve, so…"

Two minutes of silence. I wonder whether to ask about the tooth, the pain and the anaesthetic. I wait.

"I must say that after the last session I had some big problems, it was very difficult… So, regarding the uncertainty about what to do, I decided to involve my parents as well… I never do that, in fact I never talk to anyone about the sessions, only to someone I really trust, if they ask me something. I prefer not to explain, not to say that I'm in psychotherapy… I say, 'I have an appointment'."

"Perhaps saying that protects you… maybe it depends on a lack of definition of what you are doing, both for yourself and for others… it's a commitment, in fact…"

She looks at me intently, sighs, moves, changes position, looks at me again.

"I know this is the place where I can think, meditate… well, maybe even a little too much… expose my problems…"

"I meant talking to your parents. I imagine you already knew what their response would be… perhaps that's why you went there. It seems like something that tends to reduce your independence a little, as if you were afraid of making your own choice…"

"I talked about it because it was an important decision. My father gave me valuable advice, based on his experience... He is often a bit foresighted... He told me that after the blow I received, therapy cannot solve all the problems I've had in four months, but that it will take years... Maybe he's not very knowledgeable in this field, but I trust him!"

Inside, I think that the control she entrusts to her parents also refers to that over a young psychoanalytic couple at work. I think that her father's experience is a guarantee against my possible inexperience.

"It's true that you presented yourself as small, sick and insecure."

"Yes, perhaps that's true!"

"I think it's important to understand how you view the sessions. As something limiting? Something that reduces your autonomy and your freedom?"

"Why do you say that?"

"It seems to me that for you, continuing the sessions means feeling ill... On the one hand, you hide the fact that you are in psychotherapy from the world because there is a risk that they will see you differently, that is, as suffering... On the other hand, you feel you still need it, so you make yourself small and go to your parents to ask their opinion... Then here with me, you try to find reasons why it is necessary to continue. You feel good, but you also feel dependent... You want to continue, and perhaps that is why you feel you have reduced your autonomy."

Silence falls again. She seems present and thoughtful, as if she is sorting things out inside herself.

"It has always been difficult for me to choose, to have something precise and well-established, defined and not vague."

"I think that the difficulties, the struggles, the suffering of these last few sessions depend precisely on this... that is, on the fact that we are trying to define what is happening inside you, and also in these sessions... We are taking stock of what has happened and, in a certain sense, we are establishing a programme... but for the future... Things are changing... It certainly seems like the analysis is going more in depth."

She nods, absorbed and silent. And so, the session ends amid "mmhs", "ahhs" and sighs.

As a patient, I would have given my soul to read something my analysts had written about me. Not only to learn more about myself: I imagine I would have learned something more about the analysts themselves.

Then there is the other side of the coin. What is the use of all that secret material, subject to the inexorable laws of privacy, as well as the even stricter rules of professional ethics?

These are pages that are very dear to me, which, in addition to talking about patients, also tell the story of my work, my struggles, my initial efforts, my first sessions, my growth, the changes I went through, and my progressive and increasing confidence in myself and in psychoanalysis.

But they are also pages that must be protected, even destroyed, so that the confidentiality that patients know they can find is truly guaranteed forever, even after I am gone.

Paula – Friday, 10.45 a.m.

The first interview was scheduled for mid-morning. I had slept well that night, so I got up a couple of hours early to get ready calmly: I didn't know the area well and still had to figure out how to get there. I wanted to try to do things right for once.

I've always cared a lot about my appearance. Ever since I was born, everyone has told me I'm pretty, but whether I'm intelligent is anyone's guess. First things first, a nice shower. Shampoo, conditioner, body oil. Bathrobe. Hairdryer, brush, ceramic straighteners, let's straighten this hair, especially my bangs. I cared about my hair, even if I didn't act like it at the time.

Make-up. Not much, just a light touch, but effective. I wanted to look natural, but a few flaws always need to be concealed. It's difficult to erase them. Perfume is important, it's like a calling card that lingers in the air.

Finally, clothes. The hardest part. It's no coincidence that I work in fashion. That's exactly why I was in Milan: I was born in Brazil, after attending schools all over the world following my father in his appointments first as consul and then ambassador, I had expressed a desire to study industrial design, but it wasn't my road. So, I switched to graphic arts. At that time, with my family we were in London, but when I finally realised that my true passion was fashion, I moved here, where the most prestigious schools are located.

Back to that morning, I was grappling with the fateful question: what should I wear?

I had a vague idea. A cashmere jumper, simple, without a blouse underneath. Black opaque tights, mid-heel ballet flats. A skirt, without a doubt. A miniskirt, a micro-skirt in red tartan fabric. Colour combinations are essential. I liked the outfit. Maybe it wasn't practical, but my legs were on full display. They are long, shapely, and impossible to ignore. They are mine; they are me.

But then, when I was finally ready, I realised, as usual, that I was late. I had to run; I didn't want to make a bad impression on my first day.

I think I was a normal child. Perhaps somewhat neglected by my parents, that's true, but that's how the life of diplomats is: lots of social engagements, constant relocations. I was practically raised by a nanny, whom I have fond memories of, except that she used to put me fully clothed under a freezing shower when she couldn't get me to obey her.

I don't even know how many cities, countries and even continents I moved to. And it wasn't easy to start over every time: new school, new classmates, new language.

You feel like you are being constantly put to the test. And then there is the paradox of living in an exclusive, somewhat protected environment, but without any real control: what did my mother know about my thoughts and, even more so, about my sorrows? Absolutely nothing. When I was little, I missed her terribly, especially from an emotional point of view, but when I reached adolescence, the clashes began. Our relationship, which had been cosy and muffled, turned into constant conflict. Not to mention my relationship with my father. At 14, I got my first slap and then he didn't speak to me for three months: he had caught me kissing a boy, the son of friends, at a party. I was precocious, sex came early, too early, in my life. Perhaps I used promiscuity to attract my parents' attention. I remember that at the end of yet another argument, my father said to me, "Do whatever you want," and I took him literally. I didn't know the meaning of the word "limit". In the end, I didn't even know what I was doing with my body anymore.

When I arrived at the office, I hoped to rush straight into the room. Instead, there was a waiting room. I wanted to stand there, but with that micro-skirt, I didn't even know how to sit down without looking indecent, so best option was to perch on the tip of the cushion lying on the sofa.

Then he arrived. I had almost forgotten him. The reason I was there.

After that bad bout of depression the previous year, I was wandering from one doctor to another. I had started to feel anxious, then increasingly sad; at first, I had played it down, until I found myself wanting to throw myself under a train.

My mother rushed over from Stockholm and took me to New York for a psychiatric consultation. Excellent choice, good shrink, right treatment, good recovery. Not total, not totally satisfactory. Something unpleasant remained inside me. And in Milan, I didn't know who to turn to. Until a fellow student told me about this psychoanalyst, and I decided to give it a try. And here I am.

"It must have been very difficult to get here…" Not a bad start.

I thought I had prepared myself the best I could, but he caught on immediately that I was bluffing.

I had spent a couple of hours sorting out every detail, and in a few seconds and a dozen words, everything was dismantled and brought back to the core of my struggle.

I looked at him in disbelief. How did he figure it out? They call it intuition. It is based on a rapid and automatic processing of feelings, moods and thoughts.

It was a flattering experience – being understood without even speaking – but disturbing at the same time. Like feeling exposed and unprotected. I was a little scared, but immediately afterwards I breathed a sigh of relief and relaxed my muscles. I remember leaning back in my chair and starting to talk. Even today, I am convinced that that very direct opening was the cornerstone of our meeting and our subsequent work together. Raw but accurate words that I – I speak three languages fluently and understand three others – would never have been able to find. The simple truth.

"I'm throwing myself away," I began. My tone of voice was firm, but I think the doctor sensed all the despair I was hiding. I went on to tell him about my last few years: drug use and abuse (hashish, ecstasy and cocaine), lots of alcohol and just as much sex. If he really didn't want to treat me, it was better to tell me straight away.

The common thread running through my life, at least my adult life, has been seduction. And I can say with a certain amount of presumption that it had worked in that room too. Because I don't think he was dying to take care of someone like me, but I knew that after meeting me, he couldn't ignore my request for help. The net was now stretched tight; my senses had saturated his office.

Sight: an intense, penetrating gaze, curious and frightened at the same time. Irresistible.

Hearing: the acoustic plane was activated by the voice – my *child's voice* – and by the sweet lilt of my accent when I speak Italian.

Smell: I had chosen the perfume very carefully. It spread throughout the entire room, ensuring that a memory of me would remain there for a long time.

Touch: when we said goodbye at the end of the session, I made sure to leave my warm hand in his.

I spared him the sense of taste. I didn't want to win too easily. Seduction was the only way I knew to connect with others.

But I didn't want to trick him, I was afraid he would fall for it. I needed his mind to remain alert. Even though I was a little afraid of that.

I arrived 15 minutes late for our second date.

"It will never happen again," I told him as I walked in.

It was clear that I was trying in vain way to confront my limitations. Like when, after a few sessions, I said, "I want to commit myself to not drinking or taking drugs anymore."

Leaving for Milan also helped me to break off the most dramatic of a series of relationships that was always pervaded with elements of violence and oppression.

"Paula, the way you relate to the opposite sex makes me think that you cultivate such high standards and ideals that it becomes difficult to achieve them. The result is that you feel incapable, useless, disappointed. As if you were constantly oscillating between dreams of omnipotence and awakenings of impotence. It's enough to drive you crazy."

Little by little, memories, images and fantasies came to mind, relating to distant needs for care and attention. Until, when finally, I felt like even lying down on the bed in that room where tenderness started eventually replacing the erotic dimension by even in that room. Several times a week. At first, it reminded me of evenings and places of wild sex. Later, it began to seem like a place to sleep. Like a child. Freer.

That space was where I felt welcome and held, I could accept it and use it. Even in my own silence or when crying, desperate and angry. Talking about beautiful things, no longer afraid of attracting attention, or about ugly things, as if I were with another father, not the one who brought me out only to be – the daughter to be shown off in public –and only if I dressed the way he wanted.

I believe I have always paid so much attention to my body stems because the only compliments I ever received from my father were always about my physical appearance. I was a little gem, the pride of the family. And with puberty – became a real trauma given the effect my body had on myself and others – I began to replace my usual language with that of sexuality. My body instead of words.

Analysis allowed me to rediscover the oldest and most effective language, the lost language.

But at a certain point, I thought my body rebelled. I began to find it increasingly difficult to swallow food, or to perform any movement that involved repetitive gestures, such as combing my hair, an essential daily action. At first, I thought it was psychosomatic, psychological reasons, but luckily the doctor didn't fall for it. He convinced me to seek the opinion of a neurologist. The diagnosis came after a long series of visits, tests and consultations. *Myasthenia gravis.* Not reassuring.

There were many hypotheses, therapies and waiting periods. To get treatment, I had to move to Rio, where my parents were living at the time. I was starting to feel better when another blow came. I called him immediately.

"Doctor, I also have *lupus*! I can't come back. Would it be a problem if we resumed the analysis in a few months? Maybe we could stay in touch by email."

What a paradox! I, the person who had invested everything in my body, who had communicated, seduced, conquered and destroyed with my body, was forced to use only words.

My room, my place, my couch, everything or almost everything became virtual. Precious, but virtual. Virtual, but precise. Written, inescapable.

The nice thing was that he also had to write, to speak through writing, to put pen to paper.

Beginning

First, I want to say hello and tell you that I'm thinking of you and miss you. Don't worry, this isn't a declaration of love. But you were right, I've grown fond of you and you're one of the reasons I want to return to Milan. No, I haven't been drinking tonight. To tell you the truth, I have, but only one beer. I went out for sushi with my mother.

I have a question: when you write to me, you'll have to give me feedback, won't you? You can't just say nothing, or you'll probably just reply with a message saying you've received it or something like that. So how does it work? But I still like the idea of being able to stay in touch with you, even if I can't hear your voice. I think it's easier to write than to speak.

I'll tell you about my day, or rather, the highlights of my week.

Illness

Well, there are fantasies about the disease. I don't think about it so much now, but when I started researching it, I made a lot of associations. Perhaps I should also mention something that embarrasses me terribly, perhaps I've already told you about it, but I can't remember. Words embarrass me, I can use them when I'm joking, but they're monsters when I'm serious, perhaps because I'm talking about myself. But I think I must take advantage of this opportunity: when I found out I had myasthenia gravis *and had to have my thymus removed, I thought that with what had happened in Paris, it was to be expected. One evening I went to a party and ended up in bed with a guy, cute, all right. But the next morning I woke up with him on top of me having sex with my breasts and ejaculating on them. Pretty much right where they told me the thymus is. There you go. Of course, I hurt myself quite badly. Or, at least, I didn't protect myself properly. But who was I sleeping with at the time?!?*

Parents

Yes, I really think that my parents' parents weren't equipped either. The other day my mother said to me: "I hope you won't be as bitter with us as I am with my parents." My grandparents didn't let her live, or rather, they didn't prepare her for life. Those were different times. However, if I was ever angry with them, as you say, I am no longer. I think that by forgiving them, I have lifted a weight off my shoulders, and if I have children, I will only talk about the good and right things they taught me. Now my dad calls me lobinha, *which means little wolf in Portuguese. I wasn't used to this tenderness from him. The illness has changed many things between us, but above all within myself: my parents, for example, did not expect such a pragmatic reaction from me. At first, I realised they were terrified, and it was probably my calmness that began to reassure them.*

You know what? The thing I saw in my mother that I see in myself, apart from the mole near my nose, was a lack of willpower and the fact that no one had taught us how to think. And I told her: you are an intelligent woman, but no one taught you how to think for yourself, and that makes things much more difficult.

"Good morning, Paula, that's a beautiful thought you have about thinking. I have one too: I like to think that one of the things that is happening in this analysis is that you are learning to think."

Yes, I also liked this thought about thinking, and what I like even more is the fact that you think I still have time to learn.

Therapy

I like being able to think about my choice of words, to change them when they don't seem effective, although I do the same when I'm with you, don't I? But since I haven't seen you, I miss your presence, not so much you as a person, but your voice. Your voice is very important to me. In fact, I can't stand my own voice – the one others hear – because it sounds like a little girl. I often write things that I later delete. For example, I was about to delete the last sentence, but I can't do that with you, so I think I must try to write the way I speak, without deleting anything, but only adding. I hardly ever remember my dreams these days. If I do, I'll try to take notes. In the only dream I remember, I was walking down the street in Milan, thinking about how I feel when I walk here, comparing there and here. At first, I didn't really understand my feelings. I feel normal, you know fine, but now I think the question was different: where do I feel most at home?

It's strange, I sit in front of this screen for three hours (exactly the time of one session multiplied by four) and I feel like I'm saying less than I do with you in the 45 minutes we have, some of which are spent in silence. Maybe it's because writing requires more precision, or perhaps more responsibility. I don't know.

I'm fine in this city, but I miss Milan.

"Dear Paula, it seems to me that here in Milan you have found a sort of emotional home, especially after travelling so much, and not coincidentally now that you are far away."

Moon Face

My neck and face are swollen. I have chubby cheeks, as my boyfriend says. What's more, my clothes almost don't fit me, but just barely. It's not that I've become a whale, but I don't recognise my face, I look like a porcelain doll. So, you can imagine my complexes about having zero sex appeal and things like that. I'm also happy with the way I'm dealing with this physical change. I look in the mirror and don't recognise myself, but in some ways this helps me to have more confidence in other aspects in myself besides physical looks, it helps me to be stronger.

A Beautiful Old Lady

Even though I care about my appearance, even though I always wore make-up and thought about clothes and so on, I've never been obsessed with creams or other things. But with my illness, creams have become like toothpaste: I can't do without them. Well, it means I'll age better!

Speaking of illness, I think it's pretty much under control, I'm no longer in pain and my skin is also better. Every now and then I feel a little tired, but nothing out of the ordinary, I just feel like I'm out of shape, that's all. My doctor says my tests are fine and that I look like a healthy person. He even complimented me recently, saying I was a Valkyrie for the way I behaved.

Patience is a great remedy.

And it was precisely patience that allowed me to wait as long as necessary to be treated in my own country before returning to Milan, resuming my life, my relationships, my work and my therapy. It wasn't so strange to see the doctor again. The hundreds of emails and messages we exchanged during those six months allowed us to keep our connection alive. Through thousands of words, the bond held strong. Even though my body was desperately communicating illness, suffering and fatigue, our words never failed us. They were truly our "words to say it". To heal, to keep me together. I, who had made my body my reason for living, I, who received and transmitted everything I had through physical contact, had to accept to put a virtual body into play. I experienced a virtual relationship, but it was never trivial, cold or detached.

Every time we said goodbye at the end of a session, it was preceded by the same phrase: "See you next time."

I even found myself wanting to write it in emails. Better than "see you soon", more precise than "goodbye", less formal than "best regards", much closer to what I really felt and missed.

I hope you write to me soon, *pois estou com saudades.*

14 The Analyst's Illness

"Tell us, doctor, why do you want to become a psychoanalyst?" Three commissioners responsible for evaluating my application to join the Italian Psychoanalytical Society asked me this question.

"Because I am undergoing personal psychoanalysis, which is helping me to feel better. I can see that it works, so I thought I would like to practise it as a profession."

The answer was satisfactory, I think. I began and completed the *training*.

Every "sufficiently healthy" psychoanalyst knows that part of his professional choice stems from personal suffering to a greater or lesser extent. This is another reason why we must undergo analytical treatment during the training. It is not just to "heal themselves in secret" (Nina Coltart, 1993). It also serves to experience psychoanalysis first-hand, on the job, and in practice. And to know exactly what to offer the people we will meet in our work.

It is easier to follow prescriptions if trust has developed in the therapeutic relationship, allowing the patient to confide in the therapist. If the therapist has experienced first-hand what they are recommending, they are able to convey greater conviction about the appropriateness of the proposed intervention. This shared experience also helps to understand the reasons behind a recommendation.

In the film *A Doctor, a Man* (Randa Haines, 1991), a surgeon discovers he has throat cancer and, for the first time in his career, understands what it means to be ill. The long and painful process of diagnosis, acceptance and treatment of the disease transforms his attitude towards life, colleagues and patients. This leads him to include the experience of putting themselves in the shoes of a person undergoing diagnostic tests for a disease in the training of his students, medical students. To really experience what illness and treatment mean.

Then, sometimes, even the psychoanalyst gets sick. It is a difficult hypothesis to accept.

We mistakenly think we are programmed to help others, not to take care of ourselves.

Firstly, I am talking about organic illness, the kind that we, like all mere mortals, must face. We do not really know how to behave when it happens.

DOI: 10.4324/9781003759034-14

This topic has not yet been the object of thorough discussion.

What to say, what not to say, negate, up until the very end. To ourselves, first and foremost.

And then some patients, after the summer or Christmas holidays, arrive at their analyst's door and find it closed. Forever.

Almost none of us think about or give instructions on who will take care of our patients after our death, whether we are aware of being ill or it comes unexpectedly. It is therefore not surprising that it is so difficult to reflect on and discuss these issues. Who is truly capable of preparing for their own demise? Being ill, feeling mortal, dealing with other people's concerns, coming to terms with one's own end can trigger unpredictable and unthinkable emotions. Deep down, a human being can only live each day if they imagine themselves to be immortal, as if the end of life did not concern them.

But when it comes to the psyche, what happens when we must deal with "our" illness?

I remember that elderly lady, thin, with medium-length white hair, courteous and sad, whom I met in the room of the clinic where she was hospitalised. Tired and a little suspicious, she chatted kindly with me, a young doctor on night duty. Her mind was filled with dark thoughts, delusional beliefs, and obscure and threatening plots all aimed against her. She recounted them with intense emotional passion.

At the same time, she was critically aware that they were unfounded and unreal. She was very interested in my work, asking precise and competent questions that amazed me. "I'm a psychoanalyst…" she said at one point, almost ashamed. I didn't think it was yet another derailment of her thinking, but I looked at her with concern and amazement. As if sensing my thoughts, she added, "The daily struggle is to distinguish my patients' fantasies from my own…" I was struck, almost paralysed by her words.

At that time, I was immersed in the idealisation of psychoanalysis, a field that was supposed to be pure and uncontaminated, without blemish or disease. I left the room feeling bewildered. On the one hand, I appreciated my colleague's sincerity and awareness, but on the other, I wondered anxiously about the fate of the people who entrusted themselves to her.

Sometime later, I happened to meet an acquaintance of mine, who was the same age. When he found out what I did for a living, he told me enthusiastically that he had benefited greatly from therapy and shared the name of his analyst. It was the elderly lady from the clinic. I said nothing, of course. He broke the silence. "She seemed a bit strange to me at times, I didn't always understand what she was saying, but she really helped me. Thanks to her, I felt better. I remember her with pleasure and affection."

An almost unbelievable story that explains how it is easier to deal with the suffering of others than with our own, and that speaks of the mysteries of the analytical relationship and our mind.

Of course, our ability to stay in the room with our patients may be disrupted by less dramatic moments. "Are you OK, doctor? Is everything alright?" asked a patient many years ago, immediately after sitting down in front of me. It was the first session of the day. I hadn't slept much the night before. After opening the office, I rushed to the nearby newsstand to buy a copy of *la Repubblica*. I absolutely had to check that the Milan page had news of a conference I had helped organise. After eagerly leafing through the pages, having found and anxiously read the article, I took my seat at my desk. That is, maybe part of me. I was happy, but I was dripping with agitation and restlessness. My head was elsewhere. The affectionate and diligent patient noticed this immediately. I was unable to respond adequately. I smiled sadly, as if to minimise my obvious discomfort.

"Doctor, don't you ever suffer from attention deficit? How can you not get distracted?" asked a patient who had just begun an analysis with passion. Honestly interested in me and worried about herself. She's right, I thought, how can I do it?

The truth is that even psychoanalysts need help. Me too.

Pretending nothing is wrong, and denying it, being content to stay "on the right side of the table" is not enough.

Fortunately for us, there are many ways we can get help. With specific tools, such as returning to our old analyst or seeing a new therapist, seeking supervision so we can share the burdens of our profession, engaging in intervision (clinical peer reviews) with interested colleagues, attending seminars, and participating in clinical groups. Or with non-specific methods, such as practising sports or physical activities, reading books, playing an instrument, listening to music, going to the cinema or theatre, socialising with friends, travelling, cultivating hobbies, being curious, eating well and having fun in a broad sense. However, taking on management positions and roles in executive bodies or attending conferences can rarely help us with this type of problem, that is caring for ourselves.

As far as I am concerned, in addition to all the leisure activities mentioned above, I have found mindfulness to be extremely helpful as a form of "maintenance" for the mind. It offers a wide range of opportunities that are directly focused on caring for ourselves, our bodies and our therapeutic function. Because it effectively activates the delicate link between mind and body. Let me give you an example.

Some time ago, I underwent anaesthesia in the same hospital where I had been operated on ten years earlier. I remembered a particularly unpleasant phase of falling asleep during my first hospitalisation, with cold, intense tremors and fear. A specialist, who I found at the foot of my bed, witnessed my awakening which was equally unpleasant. I recognised him immediately. He had been my patient during his adolescence. He wanted to say hello and check on my condition, as I had tried to climb onto the IV stand during the post-operative period.

This second time, I feared that the experience might repeat itself, and in fact, when I arrived in the operating theatre, I began to tremble, with shivers running all through my body. Fortunately, the practice of mindfulness with breathing came to my aid. Within a few minutes, I was experiencing a completely different bodily perception: I felt as if I were being gently rocked in a giant hammock, and the shivers and tremors had disappeared. I slipped peacefully into the dormant state of the anaesthesia and woke up just as peacefully at the end of the operation. There were no trainees or former patients at my bedside.

Change of scene.

Olafur Eliasson is a Danish artist. Born to Icelandic parents, he works in Berlin. His latest interactive installation, at the Tate Modern in London, is entitled *In real life* and involves the public walking through a room/corridor full of fog. It is an experience of great emotional impact, characterised by the presence of only a few people at a time, spatial and temporal boundaries with a guaranteed visibility of 150 centimetres protecting visitors from accidentally colliding, the certainty of being able to leave and total silence. The author has defined it as a "safe space". When I walked through it, I felt very calm and at ease. I felt cautious and secure. A conscious waiting. I felt able to "linger in the experience", even enjoying features that were not pleasant at first glance.

Well, I would say that it is easy to associate this experience with some of the fundamental themes of mindfulness, such as the ability to feel, the acceptance of the moods we experience, attention to the present moment we are living and global awareness of all this.

Irvin D. Yalom, the beloved and renowned American psychoanalyst and writer, argues in *The Gift of Therapy* that relationships are paramount in treatment. Paying close attention to feelings as we experience them; learning to regularly express thoughts and emotions to patients; being able to admit our mistakes; trying to see the world as the patient sees it; developing empathy towards others; establishing a relationship characterised by authenticity, unconditional acceptance and spontaneity, a source of therapeutic effectiveness. These goals can be achieved, maintained and practised in many ways, one of which, in my experience, is meditative practice through mindfulness.

Thanks to this maintenance of ourselves, we can cultivate attention, that naked attention that allows us to be aware and therefore present in the experience of the moment, without judging it, but accepting it in its entirety.

Reconnecting with our emotions is always the primary task in healing a sick mind, while being aware of our emotions helps us to stay connected with others.

"I like it when you show how your mind works. It also helps me understand how mine works… to feel it and make it work better," a patient told me during a recent consultation.

We can heal what we can feel.

Then there is another, perhaps even more insidious illness that can affect the analyst.

It is the identity disease, the one that makes us feel that we are performing well in the room, but we are much more precarious and uncertain in our lives. And I am not referring so much to the numerous anecdotes about the distraction or vagueness of psychoanalysts, which Woody Allen has masterfully outlined, but rather to the sense of emptiness and dismay that can strike us when we leave our professional attire behind to don the more anonymous clothes of everyday life. In the room, power aside, we are invested with a role and a task that makes us feel like "someone", useful for "something". This struggle to feel "normal" must also be addressed.

Who knows whether a psychoanalyst's patient feels more at ease imagining him to be as healthy as a horse or knowing that he has also submitted himself to treatment and undergoes periodic "maintenance". Someone who seems to be perfectly "in the zone" or someone who knows their own limits? I have concluded that everyone is better off with the therapist who best matches their ideal and their needs.

15 Leaving the Room

Eleonora – Friday, 4.45 p.m.

I can't remember my first meeting with my analyst.

Many details from that period – entire days and weeks – have been lost in a blur, thanks to self-defence and, not least, electroshock therapy, which erases short-term memory. However, I remember all too well my state of mind as the hours passed slowly in the bed of a luxurious clinic where, at the age of 18, I was admitted and discharged amid the helplessness of the doctors.

What was I suffering from? The official diagnosis was "depression", and the treatments changed constantly. "Therapy," the nurse would announce in a colourless voice every time she entered my room.

I swallowed different pills all the time. But they did nothing but accentuate my impression of living in a cotton wool bubble, gripped by anxiety.

"I'm like my mother," I repeated like a refrain to every new psychiatrist who approached me.

My mother.

She had given birth to me, unexpectedly, at the age of 45. She loved me with an obsessive, stubborn love that did not permit me to stay away from her, but that didn't even let me touch her heart.

She was schizophrenic and a paediatrician, a sick woman with the authority to refuse treatment while her mind was consumed by religious fantasies and explosions of furious jealousy.

After years of trying to capture the attention of that mother and a beloved father, I had fallen into the vortex: I was convinced that I resembled her, that I was destined to lose myself in madness, totally incapable of controlling either myself or the disordered flow of events and emotions that constituted my life. The doctor worked in that clinic, and I met him in the summer.

Even today, I wonder what allowed me to trust, to put my faith in such a young doctor, who was just a "boy" at the time. He must have been in his early thirties. He looked at me, listened to me.

He wasn't afraid. And I was intrigued by his surname: where did it come from? Perhaps that was enough.

DOI: 10.4324/9781003759034-15

I must have repeated my litany to him too, I suppose: "I suffer from depersonalisation, sometimes I look in the mirror and don't recognise myself, I hear my words as if they didn't belong to me. I'm scared.".

And then tears and more tears.

At the bottom of a drawer, I find the sparse files from my hospital stays during the worst times. On those few sheets of paper, written in rounded handwriting, I rediscover his first prescription for an anxiolytic drug that remains my best friend to this day. A bit of a tyrant.

In the next file, from my second hospitalisation, I find the following note:

"Monday, 17 October, afternoon: I indicate the conditions and the contract for possible psychotherapy. She will think about it."

Thus, the treatment began, the only one that would really help me.

At first, they drove me to his office in Milan, then I returned to the clinic.

I was inert. Drained.

The first sessions were like a kind of gastric lavage: I lay down on the couch and cried. Sobbing, I desperately emptied myself of some of the anguish that was eating away at me, for which I saw no remedy.

He hardly spoke, he let me cry and, after three quarters of an hour, he said, "We'll continue next time." In a calm and vaguely questioning tone.

Then I would get up and drag myself away, wondering what we were supposed to continue, what we had ever started.

But I never missed a session.

I was always punctual, always a little early since I took the train to get to the office, on which I often fell asleep due to too many sedatives.

The doctor had set one condition: any mention of my mother, specifically the fear of madness, was dismissed. Ignored.

"We don't talk about that."

Everything else could be discussed, but, apart from that enormous anguish, nothing else existed for me. Then a difficult phase began: the pain I felt often turned into anger, into a blind hostility that made me feel like biting off the hand that the analyst was offering to me.

It was an old game; I had pushed away all my previous doctors or reduced them to impotence. I was good at it. I was strong. Stronger than them. Damn determined to defend myself, carefully guarding that pain, the only driving force that shaped my personality, my raison d'être.

Like a stray cat, I defended myself by scratching and hissing: no one would be able to get me down from the top of the tree I had climbed.

The doctor hardly spoke. I couldn't even see him, he sat behind me. I wonder if he was really listening to me. I took one step forward and two steps back, touching something of that dark *gnommero* that besieged my soul, illuminating a fragment of it, then retreating into tears. More often, into accusations. Into claims.

I made myself unpleasant. So much so that I believe that more than once he was seriously tempted to abandon me, perhaps to send me away rudely. The *peppa tencia* (pain in the neck) of the ancient card game, the queen of spades that no one wants.

"When you behave like this, there's nothing else to do but put on your raincoat and wait for the storm to pass," he once told me.

And he waited.

With infinite patience, but never passively.

He would say a few words that guided me within myself. He would hold out his hand to the stray cat so that it could sniff him and decide that, perhaps, he could be trusted. Every now and then, he would get scratched.

It is difficult to reconstruct a process of analysis.

Three times a week I lay down on that couch, in a position that never ceased to irritate me.

Slowly, I found the words again.

When psychological suffering is deep and prolonged, words get cancelled, dissolved in the acidity of anguish. It isolates you in a shapeless monad of pain that cannot be described and, therefore, cannot be understood or healed. I had to learn how to speak again, to be able to name that tangle of feelings that imprisoned me to see them better, to try to escape from the labyrinth in my mind. The doctor accompanied me, holding my hand, never dragging me, sometimes giving me a little push, but gently, delicately.

During those years, my focus in life was completely reversed. I was totally immersed in the relationship between that room and me, the doctor, the large reassuring dracaena tree opposite the couch. The world outside was a mere detail. I lived thinking about what was happening "inside", inside the room and inside my mind.

Some sessions were painful: the crying, the accusations, the feeling of not being understood returned.

He was always there. Even when I stopped the analysis.

I had fallen in love with a man much older than me. He was handsome, charming and brilliant. He made a living playing poker and betting on horses. I stopped taking all my medication suddenly, incredibly without any side effects. My natural endorphins were enough for me.

I knew it was the wrong relationship, I didn't want to analyse it, so I started leaving messages with imaginative excuses to cancel our sessions. After a month of missed appointments, I received a letter – again in that round, slightly feminine handwriting – in which he wrote that it was better to suspend the analysis for the time being, but that he, my doctor, would be there if and when I wanted to resume a conversation that was not over.

I was grateful for that reassurance and went on with my relationship, which ended two years later.

A little stronger, very bruised, I lay back down on the couch: I told him everything – he had a new office, but "my" dracaena was still there – I cried, I was not consoled. We resumed our journey.

The words now flowed more smoothly, with that full sound that a tennis ball makes on the racket in prolonged exchanges: *pof, pof, pof*, out, net and serve again.

My fears did not disappear; they played hide and seek. I was always good at hurting myself.

Well done, really. In a way, I was proud of myself.

The obsession with madness sometimes faded, giving way to other anxieties, first and foremost the terror of getting pregnant – dozens of pregnancy tests torn to pieces to see if the second line was there or not.

Then it would return.

Meanwhile, my life "outside" went on.

Years later.

One spring day, with light rain falling.

As always, lying on that now almost comfortable bed, for the first time, the doctor mentioned an event that, curiously, I had never thought about.

"Things have changed a lot. I'm sure you can walk on your own now. Perhaps it's time to start planning the end of our journey. What do you think?"

Thunderstorm, storm, strong wind.

At first, I pretended not to understand: were we going to take a break? Had I annoyed him?

Then suddenly that word, "conclusion", hit me like a slap in the face.

It meant "end".

For me, it meant detachment, abandonment.

Again, and from the very person who had saved me.

Did he make me climb down from the tree only to kick me away, treacherously?

It had been difficult to enter that room. Leaving it was even more so. I hadn't expected it.

I put up a strenuous, futile resistance. The cot had become a comfortable, warm bed. My body, made of marble, seemed unable to ever get up again.

But the doctor appeared, as always, calm, yet uncompromising: our work together was over, and the sessions would soon be discontinued.

In the end, I gave in.

I felt uprooted, torn away from that room, from the presence and dialogue with the only person who had been able to guide me without oppressing me, to help me without distorting me.

But I was beginning to realise that something important from that experience would remain: the words. The words spoken, exchanged, reborn in the intimacy of those four walls had nourished me, teaching me how to untangle the knot I still carried inside me, but which I now knew how to name, describe and therefore, at least in part, exorcise.

Yes, beyond the fear, beyond the obsessions, I was ready to leave the room.

I spent the days before the last meeting with one thought in mind: a gift.

The doctor deserved a big gift, something meaningful and eloquent, which summed up everything he had done for me and our adventure. It could have been one of the books I loved so much, but none of them were about us; or a film – he always liked them – but I couldn't choose one. Nothing was enough, nothing was suitable. I could have written a story or a long letter, but it was too soon, the subject was still too incandescent. Several times, with my typical insistence, I asked him for advice.

In vain.

"Just the thought is enough," he told me.

At the last minute, I bought a card with a cat on it, I think, and wrote these words:

If the thought is enough... Thank you for the expertise, patience and affection with which you have accompanied me through these difficult years. Take care of your beautiful dracaena and nourish it with the words that will come.

I took it out of my bag at the end of the session and placed it on the desk, this time no couch.

He asked me if he could read it right away. I was afraid.

That he wouldn't understand how true those words were. He smiled at me.

His eyelids fluttered rapidly.

"Thank you," he said to me. And I left the room.

16 At the Door… and Then

The most emotional moments of my work are the first meetings. And then the last.

So, I pay particular attention to the "farewell ceremony", the final session of therapy.

The conclusion.

A moment in which we try to reconsider the meaning of the work done.

A moment that we await with shared emotions.

A moment in which I also foresee some changes from the usual setting.

Something has changed further in recent years.

I had been treating Patrizia for a long time, a teenager with a serious eating disorder and other dystonic ailments. Things had been gradually improving; she had enrolled in medical school; she had rediscovered a reasonable harmony both internally and in her relationships. We had decided to conclude our journey. However, her parents were very concerned about the end of therapy and had asked me for a meeting to discuss it. They had accompanied their daughter's journey with discretion and respect. It was easy to reach an agreement and find common ground even at that moment. We said goodbye with affection and mutual gratitude. Once the pleasantries were over, now standing at the front door, her mother hesitated to leave, until she said to me in one breath: "May I give you a kiss?"

Before even thinking about it, before going over the rules in the good therapist's manual, I offered her my cheek. And then the other one, too.

It's not a rule, it depends on my interlocutor, it varies each time, but since then, at the end of an analysis, I let my patients decide how to say goodbye, whether with a simple greeting, a handshake, a hug, a kiss, a pat on the shoulder, a word, a gesture, a small gift, a book, a film, a CD or whatever else. And I also allow myself the freedom to decide how to respond to their greeting.

Gifts. Another recurring theme in our profession. For a long time, it was absolutely forbidden to accept any gifts from patients. There are stories of objects left on desks, waiting for who knows what, perhaps in the hope that the unfortunate patient would decide to give up the gift and take it home. Unfortunately, more perishable gifts such as flowers, plants and food have

DOI: 10.4324/9781003759034-16

also ended up there. And sadly, the humiliation of simple, genuine people who only wanted to express their gratitude has remained on those tables forever. Abandoned and misunderstood, like their gifts.

Rules should always be adapted to the situation. It is also true that no therapist should accept gifts that are overly generous or excessive, and that every action must always be considered according to what it may signify, at the time and occasion in which it occurs.

"It's the thought that counts…" is therefore a good principle. However, I fondly remember the two coffee cups received from someone who had asked me for a long time, in vain, to have a coffee together. Or the drawing and photos from someone else, an old family book, a personal object. And others too. Symbolic and meaningful. Never random. And never embarrassing.

Sometimes reciprocated, yes, I confess, in the reciprocity of a shared experience.

Because perhaps the most beautiful aspect of therapy lies precisely in the end. Right, on time, confident.

"That's fine, now we say goodbye… but if I still need you… can I come back?"

Finishing, concluding, interrupting, suspending, ending. So many ways to say goodbye.

There was a time when we lulled ourselves into the illusion that the end of an analysis, no matter how long it took, was a guarantee of achieved and definitive stability.

A long time sharing and then, suddenly, silence and mystery. Our door must close, necessarily and rightly so.

What dismay, almost a tragedy, then, to find a message on the answering machine, receive a phone call, or a request for an appointment from a former patient. A failure?

No.

Sometimes it becomes necessary to reopen the doors.

So now we can say that they have progressively become revolving doors.

Closed, but easily opened in both directions. When needed.

Now, returns are no longer tragedies or failures, but new opportunities, different needs at different stages of life. Being sought out again, establishing opportunities to meet again to check on how life is going, receiving updates on developments in life has become a way of placing our work on the plane of the possible and the real. Far from the ideal. As close as possible to normal human experience, notwithstanding the special unique relationship that is been created.

When is it necessary to return?

Why do we do it? Why return to a place that is certainly not only tiring, and to a person who has already asked and would ask again for so much in terms of commitment? Nostalgia, pleasant surprises, problems, new challenges, unexpected phases, deadlines, losses, opportunities, lost abilities, fears, births, bereavements, second thoughts, desires, everything perhaps.

The door is there, the room too. So are we. The journey resumes, or rather, continues.

Because once you have encountered psychoanalysis, it stays with you forever, so much so that the words leave the room and nestle somewhere in your thoughts, commenting on your choices. At least for some people, in a sort of internal dialogue ("we have lots of chats while I'm cycling, walking, on the underground"), someone you can always talk to, whenever you want, and not just when you open the door of the waiting room and enter the room.

Psychoanalysis itself speaks to those of us who are therapists, taking us to new worlds beyond the textbooks, changing us and opening our minds and hearts to new experiences.

17 Outside the Room

I remember quite well the last time I saw you. Alive.

It was a Wednesday evening, around eight o'clock. After seeing my last patient, I rushed to Via Tadino.

"Just a moment," Anna had said, "he's very tired."

She had welcomed you back into the house you had left a few years earlier, but which was still full of you.

Your vinyl records, thousands of them, the record player, lots of books, lots and lots of them, and memories. A painting was hung on one wall; I believe and hope it's still there.

I must tell this whole story properly. The painting is a brightly coloured acrylic, one square meter of pop art. It depicts a faceless half-bust in the act of pouring water from a kettle into a red American coffee cup. Yellow background, blue kettle, green jumper, two large pink hands. It was around 1990. I had seen it hanging on the tall, elegant wrought iron fences of Hyde Park. This, together with other works by the same painter stood out for their cheerfulness, in contrast to the typical flat London sky. I liked it immediately, it was love at first sight, but I didn't have the funds necessary for the purchase and shipping at the time. However, I knew that I would be back soon for another conference. And this time I was prepared. I withdrew money – illegally, I admit – from the family account and made the purchase on Sunday morning, a few hours before leaving. A few weeks later, the painting arrived at my home. Amazement, disbelief, a little concern about the expense – £700 – but also appreciation for the initiative and the choice. The only problem – which would also turn out to be a stroke of luck – was that the painting had been slightly damaged during transport. It was promptly replaced by another, new and slightly different one, without even having to return the first one to the insurance company.

When Gherardo saw it, he liked it immediately. He loved London, pop art, strange and original stories. A few years later, I gave him the slightly damaged copy for Christmas. We were happy.

You would be really thrilled to know that now that artist – whom I never met personally, it was her husband who sold her paintings on the street – has

DOI: 10.4324/9781003759034-17

become a star and that her works are worth much, much more. It was a good deal and a strike of excellent intuition, no doubt about it!

"Of course," I replied to Anna. I knew I would find very little of the friend I knew. You had become so small, almost shrivelled, a shadow. You recognised me, greeted me, mumbled something. "I'm dreaming, don't worry…", you said to me in response to my perplexed and confused look.

We said goodbye.

That night you left us, alone, lost, incredulous.

I have an even clearer memory of the last visit just before that evening. Luck and consolation.

The previous Saturday – I hadn't seen you for a while before then, I had only spoken to you over the phone, you had already been in bed now for a few days – in the room that had belonged to your daughter Camilla.

I walked in, you greeted me, smiled, and said, "I think the situation is out of control. I feel like in that song by Gaber, 'Quello che perde i pezzi' ['The One Who Loses Pieces']".

We had a good laugh and sang a bit of it together.

The control tower's call to Major Tom, lost in space in David Bowie's "Space Oddity", would have been fitting too. One of your favourite songs, almost prophetic.

We spent some peaceful moments together. And we managed to say goodbye properly. Without saying it.

In the same days that Gherardo passed away, Umberto Eco also left us. Claudio Magris wrote "Ricordo dell'amico scrittore" ["Memories of my Writer Friend"] in *Corriere della Sera.* His tribute concluded: "And I think of all the brotherly laughter that helps us live better." Comparing ourselves to two giants is certainly disrespectful, but it happened to us too, and I am convinced that the privilege of being able to laugh with our dearest friend (as well as talking, arguing, sharing and growing, both personally and professionally) made our lives more beautiful and made us better people.

I cannot remember the first time we met. It was certainly more than 40 years ago, in Ward II – Psychiatric Clinic, Milan General Hospital. We were interns, volunteer trainees, although in two different wards, you in the male ward, I with the women. We met during clinical discussions, supervision, exchanges, learning, training and so on. I really don't know how or why, but we became friends even before we were colleagues.

If the things I have described in the book happened in my room, it is also thanks to you.

You yourself helped make it what it is. I know there were many other moments that bound us in our special friendship: the winter walk to Buco del Piombo, immortalised by a fleeting black-and-white self-timer photo in the snow; the séance in Erba with a small table that spelled out the letters *Amici* (Friends), for which I am still unjustly credited; the trips to family homes by the sea or in the mountains; the study group in Via della Gallina – your house – on Willard Gaylin's *The Meaning of Despair*; the evenings of study groups led by Enzo Morpurgo at the Umanitaria; concerts, chats, beers, Nutella, music, Inter…

I am fond of our visit to number 1 Via Corridoni in Milan, the headquarters of the Italian Psychoanalytical Society (SPI). It was the autumn of 1978. I still remember the excitement and pride with which we entered the prestigious building, climbed the stairs to the secretary's office, and asked for a list of training analysts so that we could begin our training as psychoanalysts. Like two good brothers, we divided the names from a faded photocopy, and began a story that lasted, with ups and downs, until 2011 for you – with your resignation – and which continues for me.

The story of the SPI is also one that needs to be told.

As for all aspiring psychoanalysts, the "Society" was our goal, dreamed of, coveted and very, very painful. Personal analysis, selection interviews, didactic analysis, new selection interviews, lectures, seminars, supervision, conferences, books, studies, comparisons, discussions. Financial sacrifices, many, many sacrifices: many of us worked just to be able to pay for this adventure, this "luxury".

It was a place of great discoveries, experiences, learning, human relationships – the class group, unforgettable.

But later, little by little, it became a place of disappointment and suffering. Gherardo and I were both restless souls, a little rebellious, a little presumptuous perhaps, but in any case, curious, even too much so, intrepid travellers of the world and of the mind. Institutions, such as political parties and churches, have always been restrictive for us. We believed, sincerely, naively, generously, that we could bring some of the new things we were discovering into the psychoanalytic house we lived in. It didn't always go well. One day, Gherardo resigned. I did nothing to stop him. By then, his scientific and human interests were taking him elsewhere. Even the greatest loves can end.

Our stories often ran parallel. In May 1981, we got married a week apart. In June 1984, our daughters were born five days apart. We did a lot of things together. It is impossible to list them all, difficult to separate the professional from the personal. Perhaps there was never a real separation.

With him – I was the tutor for the Guided Practical Experiences (GPE) part of his course at Cattolica, one of the most concrete and practical aspect of teaching, a real learning experience in the field – I began my work at the university. It was fascinating to work alongside a professor who began his lessons in such a creative way, sometimes by playing songs for an entire class without commenting. My GPE, conceived and designed together, dealt with extreme freedom and inventiveness with "non-places", public services for adolescents, youth centres, therapeutic communities, sports fandom, radio and television programmes for adolescents, comics, music groups, shopping centres and anything else that seemed interesting and a source of possible discoveries and reflections. A real laboratory of life experiences and clinical practice. A window on the world.

We also held courses on the evaluation of the effectiveness of psychotherapies in specialisation schools. When we went on stage together, it was a real moment of pleasure and fun for us. We worked, taught and learned with joy.

Every now and then, Gherardo would "discover" a new source of interest, a curiosity, an experience.

Linguistic research and transcription of interviews; affective codes and thematic motifs; clinical practice and treatment, when theory was more important; empirical research; the reflective function; adult attachment; the relational shift; mind and neuroscience when it still hadn't become fashionable; spirituality and Buddhism. Finally, he was among the first to study, train, practise and teach mindfulness.

He had intrigued me so much that in 2005 I accompanied him on a retreat to Pomaia, in Tuscany, home to a renowned Buddhist centre.

We often travelled and spent holidays together. Sometimes we played tennis. We rarely played against each other; we avoided matches between ourselves and never competed to see who was better. One summer, we took part in a double's tournament at a holiday village. We enjoyed it, feeling like the Bryan twins of the ATP circuit. Despite our efforts, the match was not going well. At the end of yet another lost game, Gherardo approached me: "Explain to me why we are losing, even though we are better, more handsome and more intelligent?" It was easy to answer him. "We are losing precisely because we are convinced that we are better, more handsome and more intelligent!" We had a good laugh, ended the exchange and turned the match around.

We were different, but each was the other's best colleague, the one to whom we could safely refer any patient we couldn't treat ourselves. For many years, we never had a real scientific debate about theories, models or approaches. We felt close, even without testing it in the field. Like musicians who don't rehearse, but when they play together, they understand each other perfectly. By ear, mutually trusting.

In recent years, however, something had changed. We felt the need to share the new things we were discovering and practising, our new ways of being in the therapy room. We had discovered the pleasure and enjoyment of doing something together, even in clinical work. Gradually, with increasing self-confidence, the relationship with our patients during sessions had become more natural, human and reciprocal. We felt the need to share what we felt, more than what we understood. Being together. The core of care.

The first opportunity was reading a book on ambiguity. The subject was very dear to us. We had made authenticity our battle cry, and we felt able to express our opinions critically. We recorded a conversation we had during a summer holiday at the lake and extracted a summary from it, which we titled "Conversations on Ambiguity at the Lake". We were convinced that it would be published immediately in any specialist journal: we were decisively rejected by *Rivista di Psicoanalisi* and *Psicoterapia e Scienze Umane.* We found a home in *Setting,* but I have good reason to believe that this was thanks to a friend.

Then came the *Manuale di psicologia dinamica* [*Manual of Dynamic Psychology*], for which he asked me to write a chapter – we signed it together – on therapeutic factors. Our relationship had taken a quantum leap.

He involved me in the ReM project, a mindfulness-oriented relational psychotherapy school. He would devote himself to it completely once he left the University.

A totally innovative and creative idea, around which he had gathered all the people he admired and wanted to have close to him on his journey. Many, perhaps too many, like those who considered him their best friend. Everyone had to resign themselves to sharing him with others, without jealousy or envy, but rather with admiration for his ability to be so important to so many. And like all people of great character, he had his faults, but after learning to live with them, I now seem to have forgotten them.

The School had reached the threshold of recognition by the Ministry of Education. It would have been a magnificent example of inclusive integration of different approaches and models. An exemplary response to the many absurd ideological, elitist and sectarian divisions in psychoanalysis. We failed. Without him, it would now have no future or meaning. Even though I feel that this interrupted dream lives on in my profession every day.

With his passing, I have lost not only my best friend and colleague, but also a brother, a mentor and an inspiration for thoughts and innovations, an avid and stimulating reader. The consolation is that he continues to live in my room, in addition to those three photos of us together, placed on a shelf in the bookcase.

Every now and then, a patient who previously visited Gherardo's room comes to mine.

These are delicate moments and choices. On one hand, I am honoured and flattered that those who met him decide to work with me. Some people like to know about the special bond that united us and to be able to continue therapy with a colleague who held him in such high esteem and was his friend. On the other hand, sharing the pain of loss was too intense to cope with. Then, each person has their own story. The most touching was a woman who met him a few days before his death. When she decided to contact me, she discovered that the yellowed piece of paper with Gherardo's name on it, which she had received in a hospital many years ago, had my name on it as well. She saw it as a sign of destiny and the right place to turn to.

I also distinctly remember the last, truly the last time I saw you. You were resting in a coffin, in the study-living room of the house that had seen us together happy and peaceful in so many moments. They left me alone to say goodbye to you. You were wearing your metal-rimmed glasses – you could never be without them. We built up a rich collection of anecdotes about your visual difficulties. At the heart of your theory was the idea that disowning (or failure to recognise) was the basis of mental illness. You, of all people, who, because of your many missing dioptres, constantly feared not recognising someone.

"Pleased to meet you, Gherardo Amadei," you always said to the people we met. I always had to say, "Are you crazy? We had all just been on holiday together, at dinner last week, at that conference…" You laughed, but you preferred a gaffe to the possibility of appearing rude.

Contrite, eyes closed, you seemed at peace, finally. I gently touched your nose. It was very cold, certainly not because of the winter.

And then I felt the unbearable, definitive anger of pain.

"How can we resume that conversation we didn't finish last time?" I thought.

"We need to talk about this…" you always said, unfinished business. Leaving it in the air.

You bastard.

***

It is said that in a story nothing is false, nothing is true. In my story, every story is true, nothing has been invented, but at the same time it is false, insofar as it speaks, perhaps, of more than one person.

Some are real, others arise from the overlapping of different suggestions, they seem like a single voice, but they are a chorus, just as I heard it resonating within me, even years later.

Some people will not find themselves and may feel less important or "loved" than others. This is not the case.

Many loves remain secret, but that does not make them any less significant.

P.R.G.

Index

For Product Safety Concerns and Information please contact our EU representative GPSR@taylorandfrancis.com
Taylor & Francis Verlag GmbH, Kaufingerstraße 24, 80331 München, Germany

www.ingramcontent.com/pod-product-compliance
Ingram Content Group UK Ltd.
Pitfield, Milton Keynes, MK11 3LW, UK
UKHW020146260926
475953UK00011B/1127
9781041283539